G000016674

I'm a Patient ...
Get me out of Here ...

Self-help for
Common Illnesses

by

Dr Diana Samways MBBS

I'm a Patient ... Get Me Out of Here ...
Self Help for Common Illnesses

Copyright © Dr Diana Samways MBBS 2004

ISBN: 0-9549252-0-3

All rights reserved. No part of this publication may be reproduced, stored in a retrieval system or transmitted in any form or by any means electronic, mechanical, photocopying or otherwise without the prior permission in writing of the publisher.

Published by:

Books for Healing
PO Box 52
Haslemere
Surrey
GU27 1JA

www.booksforhealing.com

Typesetting and Production by:

Able Publishing
13 Station Road
Knebworth
Herts SG3 6AP

www.ablepublishing.co.uk
books@ablepublishing.co.uk

Unfortunately this book must carry a health warning:

If you are ill, you should see a doctor ...

However, you might like to read the book while waiting for the doctor's appointment!

The names of those mentioned in the case histories have been changed to preserve confidentiality.

Gender-sensitive personal pronouns are interchangeable throughout.

My thanks to the staff at Able Publishing for their expert and constructive input, and for the illustrations.

Searches have been undertaken to ascertain who owns the copyright to "The Velveteen Rabbit" by Margery Williams from which "The Skin Horse" is reproduced on p94. The publishers were not able to find this information in order to seek permission for the inclusion of the text but we would be pleased to acknowledge copyright in future editions of this book if the copyright owner becomes known.

Contents

Preface

"I'm Under the Doctor ... Get Me Out of Here ..."

When we get ill, we do something that is otherwise completely out of character, we take our most precious and personal possession, our body, to a complete stranger, innocently believe what he says, and then let *him take over control of our life*. Because he is a doctor we do this unquestioningly, and sometimes very expensively. We rarely feel in a position to discuss our diagnosis or the recommended treatment, let alone disagree or disobey his orders. (From which other profession do we take "orders"?) The expression "I'm under the doctor" is a reality.

Contrast our behaviour when we call a plumber to mend a broken flushing system. We discuss the options, the cost and the length of time required to fix it. As the house-owner and payer of bills, we collaborate in the decision as to whether a replacement part or a repair will be the best option. *We stay in control and make the choices.* Have you ever heard anyone say "I'm under the plumber?"

I am a conventionally trained British doctor, who has suffered considerable ill-health, and have had far too much personal experience of my own profession's misguided help, together with the powerlessness and loss of control involved. "It's for your own good." Also there is a vague feeling of personal guilt and ineptitude that accompanies being "in the sick role" as a recipient of Western Conventional Medicine.

As a result of long-term work, and some very good help, I have recovered from various common serious health problems and the results of conventional medical "treatment" and now specialise in allergy and environmental medicine, using drug-free approaches wherever possible.

This book is designed to help those people who wish to avoid being "under the doctor" and gives ideas on how they may keep control of their lives, and recover through their own efforts, with help. It is a compilation of all the various approaches that I have found useful, either for myself or for my patients. It is not meant to be scientific, as many "Alternative" therapies are difficult to prove statistically, even supposing there was money to fund trials. There are no lists of incomprehensible references from learned journals to be found at the back of this book. It contains the distilled wisdom painstakingly acquired over a medical lifetime together with some of my personal insights.

Word of mouth, clinical experience and patient recommendation are more important than trials funded by those who have a financial interest in their outcome. All the herbs, nutritional and other supplements mentioned in this book are available over the counter or via the Internet, and this is intended as a DIY manual. However it is best used in conjunction with a doctor trained in Environmental or Holistic Medicine.

The areas covered in this book range widely and my expertise is augmented, in many cases, by personal experience, so that I see many of these problems from the perspective of both doctor and ex-patient, allowing a practical and humane perspective. The subjects tackled include allergy, bowel problems, obesity, addiction and mood-swings, arthritis and many

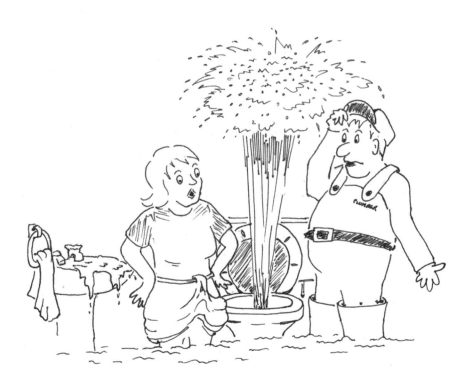

Collaborate with your doctor, as you would with the plumber ...

10

common chronic conditions, which do not yield to pills. The importance of our houses and earth energies to health, use of dowsing to sort out certain problems, the impact of mobile phone and TETRA masts and a number of excellent gadgets available via the Internet are described. The solutions offered have been found useful by myself or by patients, but have not necessarily undergone clinical trials.

There are also useful hints for coping with such intractable problems as insomnia, nightmares, apparent hauntings, the common cold and much else including maintaining health in later life and the organisation needed for dying with dignity at home. I have endeavoured to cover most of the areas which are poorly tackled or entirely neglected by Conventional Western Medicine which is very narrow in outlook, rather like looking through the peepholes in a strait-jacket.

When asked if someone should see a (conventional) doctor, the real answer (in my heart) is "no … first look at diet, lifestyle, environment etc." Sadly our medico-legal and blame industry is so out of control, that this book must carry a printed disclaimer, saying that the reader should see a doctor if they are ill … That way lies true madness.

Chapter 1

Conventional Western Medicine
The Surgeon and the Pill Fairy

As a medical student I thought that if I could know everything, cure diseases and write research papers, I would be a good doctor. Wrong. Most illness after the age of thirty-five is not instantly "curable" apart from obvious shortages (low thyroid function, for example). Most of my book is about listening to the patient and offering ones own humanity and life experience, together with some relevant education and explanation.

I do not know "everything" but I know how to find out. Someone once said "you learn more and more about less and less, and when you know everything about nothing, you graduate." Perhaps the real problem is the mental stuckness and failure of any sort of spiritual growth, that afflicts many busy doctors, lack of time being cited as the main reason.

My wise colleague, the late Dr Keith Eaton, described the process of the formation of the Medical Royal Colleges as follows:

> "First a group of senior practitioners, approaching their dodderage and who all know each other, get together over dinner and award each other a certificate which they clip from the top of a cereal packet. Having thus formed themselves into a club, which will be perceived by outsiders to be authoritative and which other practitioners wish to join, they set up an obstacle course which aspiring members then have to surmount ..."

Unfortunately there is more than a grain of truth in this, and many doctors do spend their early and busy years in practice completing the obstacle course in order to get as many higher degrees and paper qualifications as possible.

Another of my wiser medical teachers once said that medicine would be more compassionate if prior to practising, all doctors had to under undergo a major surgical operation on a British National Health Service

"Nightingale" ward (public ward for 25 people, mixed sexes, beds divided off with curtains for death and events requiring major privacy, television on at all times.) I have found that the best doctors for any particular illness are those who have suffered from it, made a good recovery and are prepared to share the relevant facts and feelings appropriately with their patients.

The River Bank Story - A Metaphor for Wisdom

There once was a wise old priest who described the three phases of his ministry.

> "I saw the people struggling with their lives, metaphorically, as people in a river, struggling to reach the river bank. At first I thought (after training) that I should stand on the riverbank and tell the people what to do and direct them by shouting instructions. Later I thought I should reach into the river, from the riverbank, and try to guide them to the edge. Much later, when I reached the age of wisdom and experience, I realised we were *all in the river together,* helping each other along."

Very few doctors ever reach this stage of wisdom, far too many behave as if they think they are God.

Riverbank Story, Two

This illustrates our current obsession with fixing each problem with the latest pharmaceutical magic bullet, without ever stopping to think about causes and future prevention. (A bit like the drug addict sorting the problems from his last "fix" with the next identical "fix" and expecting a long-term improvement.)

A group of friends were picnicking on a riverbank, when someone noticed a baby floating down the river towards them. They fished it out and dried it and generally sorted things, and were just wondering what to do, when another baby was noticed floating down the river ... they fished it out etc. etc. This continued to happen, and they got very skilled at saving drowning babies. After a while, one of the group said "why don't some of us walk up-stream and see if we can *prevent these babies from falling in."*

13

Wisdom or "Evidence Based Medicine" Can we have Both?

Our leaders insist on "Evidence-Based Medicine" to the exclusion of all else. Much of my work in the Allergy and Addiction field is based on accumulated wisdom and experience (mine and other people's) and the results are not easily quantifiable by clinical trials. Many patients come to me in despair having had "evidence-based medicine" fail them, and even make them worse.

Years ago, as a result of the witch-craft trials, a great deal of accumulated wisdom was lost, including knowledge of the correction of adverse earth energies, and their relationship to underground water, which may affect houses and cause ill health. The purpose of stone circles may be related to this aspect of lost knowledge, and certainly water dowsing is. The latter, while always considered suspect and certainly unexplainable, survived as it was the cheapest way of finding drinking water. (And it often still is.) Old churches are usually sited and orientated on especially favourable places from the earth energy point of view, which makes worshippers feel better. These sites can only be found by dowsing, even now.

It would be a pity to throw out the baby with the bathwater, again, just because a number of huge vested interests like to tell us that, if we can't count it or measure it, then it hasn't happened. We can not measure either pain, misery or wellness, let alone degrees of improvement, on any scale of units, as yet.

Often an early alert to things going wrong is given by a number of sufferers from some new syndrome or disease trying to inform the media and the medical profession. Their reports are initially dismissed as "only anecdotal" and therefore not "scientific" so they didn't happen ... (but they did). The first few cases of the plague were anecdotal, at what statistical level does something become "real"?

Recent examples of this include the MMR Vaccine and Attention Deficit Hyperactivity Disorder Controversy (Chapter 8), illnesses occurring near TETRA and other mobile phone masts (Chapter 7 and Appendix 4), clusters of cancer and leukaemia near high tension power lines, Gulf War Syndrome (Chapter 8) and much else.

The standard bleat from the big industries concerned is that "there is no evidence that ... (our expensive little wonder) ... has caused any health problems." Leaving aside that it is unlikely that they did any valid tests, it is not possible to prove a negative (that something *doesn't* happen) only that something *does happen*.

Modern Medicine is "drug firm" driven, always seeking chemical solutions to human problems. For example, there are many complex and expensively researched pills for raised blood pressure, which effectively lower it (with or without unfortunate side effects for a condition in which, originally, the patient did not feel ill). But this begs the question of why the blood pressure was raised in the first place (alcohol, tobacco, stress, weight, lifestyle, mineral and vitamin deficiencies and house problems are all possibilities) and really fails to cure anything. Good medicine tackles causes rather than offers quick fixes.

There are many health foods, supplements, vitamins and herbs which are useful in the sort of Environmental Medicine that I practise. Some are ancient knowledge (Hawthorn for raised Blood Pressure) and others are more recent discoveries. They rarely have side effects. Politically this approach is unpopular with the vested interests because these products are cheap and usually can not be patented. Some are closer to foods than to drugs.

Next we are told that because no clinical trials were done, they can not be proved to work (so they don't work ... but they do). However there is little profit in these relatively cheap products, so no-one will fund a clinical trial. In the European Union this is being used as the lever to ban herbs and nutritional supplements, by insisting on eliminating all those which have not undergone such trials, and most of them haven't. One is more likely to be struck by lightning than suffer ill-health from taking food supplements. (This avoids discussion of the hundreds of thousands of people, who, every year suffer ill-health and death from pharmaceutical preparations, which the drug companies would like to promote once they have rendered the herbs and supplements unavailable or illegal (Chapter 17 and 18).)

I am unhappy about the validity of double blind "independent" clinical trials so beloved of the drug firms and academics. These have to be funded. How can he who pays the piper *not* call the tune? We will never know how many results from clinical trials were *not* published because they failed to produce the "right" results. Very little human endeavour is truly unbiased. Behind every statistic there's a vested interest.

Recently there was a move to insist on publication of unsuccessful drug trials to redress this balance. I can't see this happening other than as a discrete list at the back of some obscure publication that is unavailable to the general public.

Clinical trials only compare a group ("cohort" is the in-word) taking one thing or pill, with an unmedicated control group. There must, however be a multitude of other variables which are not considered, not the least of which are the expectations of those involved in financing the trial.

Since writing this, I have read a book called *Seeds of Deception* by Jeffrey M. Smith. The lengths to which the big battalions will go to get untried foods and inadequately tested drugs onto the market is breath-taking and can only be described, in some cases, as fraudulent.

Drug manufacturers often do not deliberately produce drugs to fill an identified need or gap in the health market, rather they employ people to produce novel molecules and then try to find something the new molecule will "cure" (Alice in Blunderland). So we have several hundred similar arthritis drugs, with similar side effects, and still nothing effective against the common cold. They also try desperately to find new uses for "orphan drugs" (drugs which have been costly to develop and failed in their original purpose, perhaps through unwanted effects). Thalidomide and AZT are examples, the latter was eventually used as an anti-Aids drug in those with symptom-free HIV, many people are still trying to avoid it. The former was for morning sickness which produced major birth defects in babies when taken by pregnant mothers, efforts have been made to sell it for other purposes.

Almost all illness acquired in life has a major environmental and lifestyle component, and unless we deal with this aspect, neither genetic manipulation nor chemical annihilation will be curative.

The major health improvements which have occurred during the last hundred years or so have been largely due to improvements in sanitation and public health including the invention of drains and an understanding of the connection between epidemics and drinking water contaminated by sewage. In 1851, Dr John Snow stopped a cholera epidemic in London by using local knowledge and sensible observation (which would today be denigrated as unscientific and anecdotal). He removed the pump handle from the pump at Broad Street, the water from which was contaminated and there were no further related cases of cholera.

What Doctors are Good At

In general, acute infections are best treated conventionally with antibiotics (but see below), as are hormonal shortages such as an under-active thyroid (but see also chapters 11 and 18 on the menopause and natural hormone replacement therapy). Hip and some other joint replacements are a very successful way of curing arthritis pain, but they do not last for ever and may have to be redone. Also there are people who have wound up with multiple (different) joint replacements, which suggests palliation and that there is an underlying process destroying joints (perhaps mould or food allergy) which is not being tackled.

Conventional medicine is good at accidents and emergencies, fractures and repairing things mechanical, removing tumours and sorting out obstructions and blockages, hernia repairs, etc. Most of these are acute conditions and require surgery.

I have to admit that alternative approaches do not always work with raised blood pressure. In view of its tendency to cause various arterial and organ damage, it does seem sensible to reduce blood pressure with the smallest possible dose of a pharmacological drug, and monitor it at home using a self-take blood pressure machine, while seeking the cause and improving lifestyle. I do not think pharmaceuticals are wisely used as a substitute for lifestyle changes. A small dose of a beta blocker fits the bill. The more sophisticated drugs sometimes have very sophisticated side effects. Minerals (in liquid form) and vitamins, especially the B group, should be tried for a minimum of two weeks, if possible, before resorting to medication.

What Doctors are Not Good At

Most chronic physical illness, especially occurring over forty years of age, is better looked at through the kaleidoscope of Environmental Medicine in an effort to remedy the causes, and there is usually more than one cause. Chronic or recurrent infections are usually treated with multiple courses of antibiotics without any thought for their effect on the normal bacterial inhabitants (good bugs) of the large intestine which are instrumental in digestion and well-being. These latter are killed off indiscriminately and the resulting imbalance is caused by the increase in numbers of yeasts, which take up the space vacated by the "good bugs" killed by the antibiotics. They may cause major ill health, often years later. The connection is missed because of the time delay, and the fact that most doctors are totally unaware of the problem, which is difficult to "prove." (Chapters 3 and 4.)

If, dear reader, you only take one thing from this book, let it be this: *never take antibiotics without taking an Acidophilus (lactobacillus or similar) food supplement simultaneously*, and for a further week or two after the antibiotics are finished. They will replenish the "good guys" the antibiotic is going to kill off, and prevent further ill health in the future.

If multiple courses of antibiotics are required, the cause is probably not bacterial, and is an infection of a kind that does not respond to antibiotics, usually a yeast (candida) or virus infection.

Doctors are not good at allergies other than the acute life threatening kind (from say, insect stings or nut allergy requiring emergency treatment) and treat asthma with steroid (hydrocortisone derived) drugs which damp down but do not cure the problem. They routinely avoid inquiring into what is causing the allergic reaction. Most other allergies (chronic food, mould and chemical sensitivities) are entirely missed, or worse, treated with tranquilisers as the symptoms may include anxiety.

Doctors are also poor at treating addiction, which they either miss or band-aid inappropriately, usually with tranquilisers or antidepressants. When this does not work, they refer the unfortunate person to a psychiatrist, who changes the pills to no good effect. Giving pills to an alcoholic changes nothing, it will only make him smell better. And this, dear reader is the second thing I hope you will take from this book: *Insist that the alcoholic (person with a drink problem, if you prefer) goes to Alcoholics Anonymous.* Tell your GP of this apparently well-kept secret; AA is by far the most effective resource for treating alcoholism (AA headquarters has even done surveys to show this statistically, although obviously anonymously and without a control group). This subject is discussed in detail in chapter 10.

Intervention is usually possible for any chronic life problem, if the causes are tackled *at a time of crisis*. This requires skill and consultation time, and the wisdom not to "band-aid" with pills or temporary solutions, such as persuading Social Services to pay off the electricity bill which just frees up other money for buying more booze, gambling or whatever is the problem. It is vital to provide support for the patient to enable him/her to work out a lasting solution involving real change.

Finally I have concerns about treating cancer with drugs or radiation that are designed further to depress the immune system, when we need the latter to be in the best possible fettle to fight cancer and other environmental assaults. In spite of the huge sums of money spent on research; treatment of most cancers has not improved very much in my medical lifetime, and I am not sure that the pharmaceutical vested interests are barking up the right tree.

In 50 years we may well look back with horror at our present brutal methods (possibly muttering such words as "crimes against humanity"), much as we now wonder how purging, cupping and leeching can ever have had any beneficial effect, other than to the income of the medical profession and the suppliers of leeches. Unofficial rumours suggest that when cancer specialists themselves get cancer, they do not usually go for the rays and poisons approach that they enthusiastically embrace for their patients.

There are alternative approaches, but it takes courage to say "no" to the rays and poisons, and go elsewhere. Having seen friends who have had multiple courses of the radiation and chemicals, I have been struck by the feeling that there was "no-one at home" and that these people have somehow been deprived of all their positive energy and humanity. (One could say they would have been dead without the treatment, so I leave the reader, as ever, to form their own conclusions.)

How to Use Your Scientifically Trained Doctor to Your Advantage

Doctors can be very useful, provided *you keep the control*. So:

1. Decide, ahead of time, what you want from your doctor (tests to exclude cancer, or a serious blood problem, etc.) always ask for a thyroid function test when having other bloodwork.

2. If you know the diagnosis, learn all you can about your illness, (Internet, self-help groups, public library, see Reference Section at the end of this book)

3. Make a list of relevant questions, learn them but do not take the list into the consultation which will make the doctor despair if he is time-driven. (No, he shouldn't be, but British Medicine is.)

4. Review question 1 in the light of the knowledge you have gained from the research you have done, decide what you want, or want to know, ask how long it will take, what it will cost etc. (Remember the plumber at the beginning?)

Go for it (politely and with humour,) but *you* keep the control and make the decisions. Remember your GP is "not Daddy." If you are over fifty, forget that childhood scenario when the house used to be purified, and soap and clean towels were ceremonially laid out prior to a doctor's home visit. He is not God.

If referral to a specialist is being considered, choose a young consultant if you want cutting edge technical expertise and science, and an older more experienced one if you want humanity and empathy. Never undergo treatment by someone you instinctively do not like or trust or who seems to be depressed.

Avoid having medical tests or investigations *unless the results will be of use in deciding future action.* For example if there is no practical cure, the only purpose of doing tests might be organisational (of future life) rather than medical. Where tests are being paid for, question their necessity by asking "what will this tell us and what will we able to do about it when we have the result?"

Finally never have medical procedures that are not absolutely necessary for health, and ask the specialist "what will happen if I don't have this done?" Unlike television soaps, real doctors are not gods, things can go wrong or the results may not be as good as expected. To give an example: varicose vein operations are not always a total success, one might sensibly have surgery if the condition is painful, causing leg ulcers or swelling, but not, in my view, for cosmetic reasons alone.

Differences between the British NHS and American Systems

There is not a lot, but basically, the British system is rationed by time (delay and waiting list system) and the American System by money (complicated insurance set-up). The philosophy is similar but seems more drug-firm and financially driven in the USA, where there is direct advertising of drugs to the public on TV ("ask your doctor to prescribe our expensive little cure-all for you ..."), and a heavier accent on physical check-ups for early detection of illness. Also there is a direct link between the doctor's salary and the number of operations or treatments he carries out. The American public seems to have an even greater misplaced reverence for doctors and faith in their utterances than does the British, as exemplified by the many TV advertisements for dubious products from drugs to household rubber gloves, which are given the endorsement "as used by doctors."

The main difference is that in Britain you are under the care of a family doctor (GP) and in the past he would have treated several generations of the family and practised a more rounded form of Medicine than is usual today, when little can be accomplished in a five minute appointment. My mentor in General Practice once said that the GP is analogous to the conductor of a symphony orchestra, who may not play any of the instruments but he knows what they all can do and how to use them to good effect. He likened this to his detailed personal knowledge of the local specialists, and their skills.

In America people seem able to walk into any specialist's office without much guidance, and family practitioners (GPs) are not universal. However, in both countries there is an expanding market in Holistic Therapies of various kinds, and in Environmental and non-drug approaches to treating illness successfully.

Chapter 2

There is an Alternative Way - Holistic Medicine

There is a relatively small number of doctors who practice Holistically, they are often Allergy Specialists or Nutritionists and may use the expression Environmental Medicine in describing their work. They mostly practice privately as the NHS does not yet embrace this approach despite the savings of millions of pounds that could be achieved by the reduction of expensive drug prescribing and complications therefrom. (Unfortunately the NHS is in bed with the drug companies.)

A doctor practising Environmental Medicine (which is what I shall call it henceforth, including allergy work and Holistic approaches) will set up an appointment lasting at least one hour, and will spend time taking a careful history of the problem in an effort to find out the causes, he will not interest himself with addressing detailed individual symptoms and "organ recitals," but will try to get an overview of the situation. He will work rather like Sherlock Holmes. When I see patients I use my expertise and experience to make a diagnosis of the nature of the problem, and then teach the patient the principles of nutrition and avoidance of allergens (environmental control) using information sheets which can be taken and studied at home. Those parts which are relevant to that particular individual are highlighted.

Patients are asked to keep a food diary for a week prior to their visit, and include all food and drink, the weather and severity of any symptoms that vary (joint pain, bloating, mood swings etc.) This is primarily designed to help them to think about any foods which may be causing problems, but is helpful to me at the diagnostic level. I encourage them to continue with the food diary for a few weeks, as they will learn from it.

This sort of consultation will not cure them in one sitting, but will give the patient back the control over their life, if they are prepared to make the dietary and other changes suggested. They will find they understand the relapsing nature of the problem, and how to prevent it, and to make an informed decision as to whether, say, that portion of chocolate chip ice cream is really worth the bloating and pain that may follow in the night or next morning.

It is important to keep the approach non-judgmental, patients have usually been excoriating and blaming themselves for years for giving in to their food cravings, not realising that allergy and addiction are two faces of the same coin (Chapter 12). It is a question of consequences rather than "sin". Many people suffer from obesity that has failed to respond to a variety of diets. They know the calorific value of everything. They often find that weight loss is a by-product of food allergy treatment, or of tackling the cause of their Irritable Bowl Syndrome, and restrictive diets involving long-term hunger and deprivation are not needed.

A good Environmental Medicine Specialist will pay attention to the patient's house and work environment. I find houses particularly important, and patients do not usually get completely well, while living in an unhealthy house (see chapter 5, 6 and 7). Happily I have not, so far ever had to recommend a patient to sell their house, although I was glad to hear that one young man was planning to leave an excessively mouldy basement flat he was renting. Most houses can be "healed" along with their owners apart from the visibly mouldy ones, where the moulds probably produce an airborne toxin (poison) as well as the allergens.

Environmental approaches aim to strengthen the patient's immune system, general health and resistance. When orthodox doctors consider infection, they think of bugs and antibiotics, but never of "increasing host resistance" by improving nutrition. A healthy diet, including "food combining", and nutritional supplements are vital, as are decoding packaging labels to understand what the manufacturers are adding to food items. Much food is now so over-processed as to be nutritionally valueless, other than as entertainment for the taste buds. Microwave ovens kill the "life-force" in food, and, personally I only use them very occasionally in emergencies.

Irritable Bowel Syndrome and many allergy problems can be effectively treated in a single consultation, if the patient is motivated to make changes. They should be warned that they may feel worse ("Herxheimer or die-off Reaction", see chapter 4) before improvement, but this is a good sign that the approach is correct.

Problems which should be Treated Environmentally

Food Allergies, Yeast, Mould and Candida
Chronic food allergies are pretty well accepted, but the associated problems of intestinal yeast overgrowth and inhaled mould allergy are often missed.

Irritable bowel syndrome, joint pains, mood swings and obesity (despite dieting) respond poorly to conventional medicine (Chapter 4).

Houses and Geopathic Stress

Certain geological configurations including the crossings of underground streams at different depths may cause problems in some houses. Research in Germany in the 1930's has shown the existence of "cancer houses" where successive owners of certain houses developed cancer due to prolonged sleeping over such a crossing. Electrical effects due to modern wiring, high tension cables and mobile phone masts, including TETRA, may add to this. (Our houses are effectively Faraday Cages, animals reared experimentally in the latter fared poorly (Chapter 7).)

The Immune System and "Total Load"

It is important to minimise stress on the immune system, and one huge area of stress comes from our family of origin, especially if there was violence or other upset in childhood, including parental alcoholism. This sort of chronic fear weakens the immune system and the resulting illness usually shows up in mid-life. In addition to dietary and environmental measures, these people may need to unravel some of their childhood trauma, which was not their fault, and learn to establish proper inter-personal boundaries, avoid being sucked into other people's emotional baggage and "undo" the old destructive messages about never being "good enough" (Chapter 10).

Chapter 3

Importance of a Healthy Digestive System for Good General Health

A very high proportion of our daily energy out-put is used in digesting our food, the purpose of which is to provide the body with energy and building blocks for the processes necessary to keep us healthy and happy. It is important that our digestive system should be healthy and the food we eat should be nutritious, uncontaminated and fresh enough to contain energy or "life-force."

Our intestine (digestive tube) is about thirty-six feet long neatly coiled up. Digestion starts with the mouth, and the alkaline saliva with which food is initially mixed when we chew. Special enzymes (digestive chemicals) are added and begin the digestive process for carbohydrates. The stomach provides acid, and this is followed by bile from the liver and gall bladder and juices from the pancreas, which all aim to break down our food into manageable molecules.

The remaining thirty-three feet or so, are involved with absorbing (taking into the body) the nutrient building blocks that have resulted from the digestive breakdown process. The inside gut lining is folded upon itself almost infinitely to produce a vast surface area. The final six feet of intestine is the colon, which, I am reliably informed contains at least two pounds weight of bacteria. One would rather not dwell too much on how they arrived at this conclusion, but from a practical point of view it is very important. Among other things, the colon reabsorbs (takes back into the body) most of the fluid that has been used in the digestion process.

What Doctors Don't Tell You about Digestion and Nutrition

The nature and proportion of the constituents of this bacterial population is vitally important to our general and intestinal health and mental outlook. (See chapter 4 on Irritable Bowel Syndrome.) The main purpose of these bacteria is to breakdown cellulose and indigestible items in the diet, they may also have other functions to do with a feeling of well-being and synthesis of vitamins. For simplicity, I divide these bacteria into good bugs and bad bugs, although most of the bad guys are only bad because there are too many of them, and they are breeding out of control. These are the yeasts and candida organisms related to moulds and similar to those that cause vaginal thrush and much else.

The scene can be viewed as an organic garden where there is a natural balance of weeds and flowers, one would never eliminate all the weeds, but they are kept in check. Putting weed killer (taking antibiotics) tends to kill everything but the most hardy (in this case the candida and yeast) which then over-run the garden. See page 36 for illness and lifestyle factors that encourage overgrowth of yeast, causing intestinal candidiasis. This is sometimes known as Gut Dysbiosis, as there may be other organisms involved, although they all respond to the anti-candida diet (see chapter 4).

The Hay Diet (Food Combining) and Why it Works

The Modified Hay Diet

This is helpful for those with energy loss, wind, bloating, candida also food and mould allergies, weight problems and arthritis. It reduces fermentation of the intestinal contents which is the cause of some of the symptoms.

The mantra is: *"Don't eat Carbohydrate (starch) and Protein at the same Meal"*.

Do not combine: meat, fish, eggs and cheese (protein) with wheat (bread, pasta), oats, potato or rice (carbohydrates) *at the same meal*. It is non-restrictive in quantity, but the content is organised differently.

Don't Eat Proteins	with Carbohydrates
Meat	Wheat/oats
Fish	Potatoes
Eggs	Bread
Cheese	Pasta
	Rice

The following can be eaten with anything: All salads and vegetables (apart from potatoes) fruit, nuts, beans and legumes.

This version of the Hay Diet is used by me personally and is recommended to my patients. The original Hay Diet was more complex in

26

detail, which made life socially difficult. The main purpose is to prevent gut fermentation (gas formation) which this simplified version does.

A decision must be made ahead of time whether a particular meal will be protein or carbohydrate.

Hints

Breakfast may require creative flare, especially if yeast is temporarily being avoided, as in the anti-candida diet (page 38). The following ideas may help:

Yeast Free Carbs:

- Microchips (quick but not suitable for every day, as they probably lack any nutritional value)
- Rice Biscuits (resemble polystyrene but come in various flavours)
- Soda bread, to avoid yeast. This can be bought at Marks & Spencer and Waitrose as Soda Farles (they also do Potato Farles). Some of these items are not too sound nutritionally but can be used on a short term basis. Proper soda bread from an independent baker is better. Ready made filo-pastry (Waitrose) can be pre-cooked by folding into squares and baking, they keep crisp for days on a plate (and probably go soggy in a tin).

In the USA avoid bread made from "enriched flour" which has synthetic B vitamins added (after having been taken away, originally) these vitamins or some other added ingredient, can cause allergy symptoms in some people. Instead use those brands of brown pita bread to which synthetic vitamins have not been added, or organic sourdough (un-yeasted) bread.

Organic foods are, in theory good, however it is important that they are locally grown and recently harvested. Organic vegetables that have travelled for days without fungicide, will be mould infested and have little life-force or nutritional value. Locally delivered veggi-boxes are ideal.

When eating out, the Hay principles can be followed by having a meat or fish protein meal and almost everything else except bread, rice, pasta and potatoes.

Avoid food that has been industrialised and has become a "commodity". The ingredient list on some foods reads like an advanced chemistry textbook, see appendix 3 for translation of the disguises under which common undesirable food ingredients are labelled and divided up. Worse still are the farming practices involving chemical fertilisers, pesticides, and genetic modification. Their purpose is to sell a branded weed-killer or to delay the moment when the product goes visibly bad. This is called "increasing shelf-life" but is really reducing any possible food value or life force. The multi-nationals have quietly bypassed nutrition in favour of entertainment, and the public assumes that because a food tastes good it must be healthy. However the artificial flavouring industry can transform anything.

Other practices which reduce food value and may have unexpected long-term consequences, include hormonal and antibiotic treatment of livestock and the feeding of dead animals (including, in some countries euthanased dogs and cats, fallen cattle with diseases of unknown origin, cattle unfit to eat, and road kill) to farm animals and poultry as feed rendered into protein pellets. Even worse is the deliberate inclusion in animal and poultry feed of chicken feathers and animal faeces and much other domestic and industrial waste, the details of which do not bear thinking about. (See Fast Food Nation in the bibliography section of appendix 1, or the Internet for more on this.) Cattle are ruminant herbivores (grass eaters) and not designed to eat meat, let alone the residue of their own kind, as cannibals. It is also questionable whether cattle should be fed on grains. Most are except those whose meat is specifically marked "grass fed."

Our governments and the food multinationals are conducting a massive uncontrolled experiment with our food, and BSE (mad cow disease) is just one result of this. I am concerned that we may be mutating and spreading new viruses (for which we have no cure) though these malpractices, quite apart from severe bacterial infections, often antibiotic resistant. Campylobacter infection from chickens is a fairly recent addition to the list of common food-borne infections now affecting us.

More recent "advances" involving treatment of cows with genetically modified growth hormone to increase milk-yield have not undergone proper safety testing. The genetic modification of food is for the benefit of the multinationals, to make it resistant to the maker's own weed killer (weedkiller-ready Soya Beans) or to make it keep longer (shelf-life.) The longer food is kept the less of the "life force" or vital energy remains. Genetic modification is going to make things impossible for people battling food allergies and their doctors.

Most Americans do not realize that at least 75% of the food they buy at the supermarket in the USA contains genetically modified (GM) ingredients, or has eaten genetically modified feed-stuff. This is because their media, the multinationals and the Food and Drug Administration (FDA) have orchestrated a loud silence on the subject. The list of foods involved includes soya products, corn, certain tomatoes and potatoes and much else.

Such safety testing as has occurred, has been unsatisfactory and was carried out by the multinationals making the product concerned. Many of these trials were *specifically designed not* to show up any problems (by such devices as shortening the trial, or not looking at parts of the experimental animal that would show adverse post-mortem changes.) J. Smith's book "Seeds of Deception" says it all.

Experimental and farm animals, given a choice, avoid eating GM products, and in some experiments the product (tomatoes) had to be mulched up and force-fed to rats by stomach tube, as they refused to eat it. Since it is impossible, with bulk shipping (so they say) to keep a genetically modified product separate from a standard one, most items such as corn and soya are, in the USA, a mixture of both GM and non-GM. That means that the products made from them will contain both, this includes bread, edible oils and anything made there-from and exported to Europe.

It was decided not to label genetically modified products, as such, because it was rightly feared that the public wouldn't buy them. For the same reason, the multinationals have also tried (and largely succeeded) in preventing the labeling of foods that do *not* contain GM ingredients as "GM free." The only way to avoid GM foods in the USA is to eat organically produced food.

Irradiation is another convenience for the manufacturers and will enable them to increase shelf life and get away with increasingly unhygienic practices. Once irradiated, food has no life force and is nutritionally useless to the body. Recently blood tests were taken from children fed irradiated food and abnormal blood cells were found. Their blood count did eventually return to normal, but this is not an experiment I would wish to carry out. Originally it was decided in the USA to label irradiated food with the weasel-words "Cold Pasteurisation," but I fear even this may have been abandoned. In the UK the most likely foods to be irradiated are herbs and spices.

Recombinant Bovine Somatotrophin is the smart name for an American branded genetically engineered bovine growth hormone now given to cows in the USA to make fewer cows produce very much more milk. It is so devastating to health that the cows have a short life and develop mastitis, (udder infection leading to pus in their milk,) and require routine treatment with a variety of antibiotics, which also end up in milk and dairy products.

As yet Europe has resisted this development, however organic milk, preferably obtained from the farm from a Jersey or Guernsey herd is much healthier and tastier. There may well be a special health factor in unpasteurised milk that is destroyed by pasteurisation, and this factor may account for the astonishing view held by some doctors that the modern allergy and asthma epidemic is due to our houses being "too clean". The reality may be that children brought up on "dirty" farms drank raw milk.

Soy Products are being touted as "good for us" and are widely used in infant feeds. These are very oestrogenic, (female hormonal) and there is some evidence that they may cause breast and thyroid cancers in women and premature puberty in girls, sometimes before the age of three. Since the world is getting more oestrogenic from toxic wastes, adding to it by eating soya products seems risky. One hardly dares think what this oestrogenic substance in infant feed is doing to baby boys. Incidentally Buddhist monks who were celibate used to consume Tofu (a soya product) specifically to *reduce libido*. There is considerable recent anecdotal evidence from the USA that soya products cause under-activity of the thyroid gland.

Mechanically Recovered Meat

In order to maximise profit, it is standard slaughterhouse practice to subject the bones and other parts remaining after normal butchery, either to a high-pressure hose or to a boiling process, to remove any low-grade meat that remains. The resulting slurry of meat and water is then dehydrated into a paste that can be hidden in anything (from baby food to burgers) which is not a whole "lump" of some size. Chicken nuggets also come under this category, and some chicken Kiev is constructed this way.

There are several problems with mechanically recovered meat, apart from hygiene, these include a tendency to add parts of bovine anatomy one would rather not consider as food, including hooves, ears and genitals (ground up). However the real problem is the danger of contamination with the BSE organism. In the UK, after slaughter, the head and spinal cord of cattle are removed first and set aside, prior to butchering the animal. It is almost impossible to remove the cord cleanly and intact, so some cord contamination of the surrounding bones (spinal column) is inevitable. Even hosing down is not going to prevent the organism getting into the resulting mechanically recovered meat, and it is not destroyed by heat.

In most other countries where BSE has not yet been diagnosed, but whose rendering and feeding policies may have been similar to those in the UK, no effort is made to remove the cord, and the slaughter-lines are often run at a speed too fast to allow of such luxuries. Faecal contamination of meat is also inevitable, and as someone else so aptly said "burgers contain shit and milk contains pus."

Causes of BSE

The UK government official line is that BSE is caused by a prion protein, an as yet unidentified particle, which eventually "infects" the brains of cows, humans and some other animals as a form of brain disease called Creutzfeldt Jacob Disease (CJD.) The disease acquired from beef consumption is known as new variant CJD (vCJD) and is somewhat different from CJD which is a rare and long recognised brain disease occurring sporadically.

The prion's survival is said to have resulted from a change in the sterilisation practices involved in treating the bone meal and other animal effluent used in making high protein cattle feed pellets. A reduction in sterilisation temperatures was instigated in the nineteen eighties in order to cut production costs, and it is thought that this allowed the organism to be fed back to ensuing generations of cattle, thus causing the disease.

However the countries worst affected by this outbreak were those where compulsory treatment of cows with organo-phosphate pesticides to the skin took place. There is a considerable weight of evidence to suggest that this may be part of the cause, perhaps by lowering the cow's disease resistance by its toxicity. (Many farm workers became ill after dosing animals with organophosphate insecticides, which are otherwise used as nerve gas and defoliants in times of war.)

The person who did much of the work on this subject has had a difficult time, probably because of the huge vested interests in avoiding any public exposure of the pesticide theory and the damages claims that would ensue, as the government made pesticide use compulsory.

My Personal Food Rules

- Nothing irradiated, hormone treated or genetically modified.
- No meat that is not visible as a piece (i.e. as a limb, steak or joint), no bought mince, ground beef, burgers, sausages, salami or nuggets. (Danger from mechanically recovered meat, BSE and faecal contamination.)
- In the USA, no milk, cream or eggs unless certified organic.

- Nothing with too long a list of obvious chemicals.
- No Soya products (unhealthy and genetically modified in USA).
- No margarines or vegetable oil, except extra virgin olive oil and coconut oil (and dripping collected from home cooked organic beef, lamb or chicken for cooking). Butter in moderation.
- No sugar (honey and maple or date syrup are fine.).
- No farmed fish (the pesticide used to control fish lice is toxic, and if you ever fly over a fish farm, the water can be seen to be filthy over a wide area around the cages). Think where fish comes from, the seas are becoming very polluted with heavy metals and other industrial waste, wild Pacific salmon may be best.

One of the few advantages of the vastly expensive European Union is that our food safety rules are stricter than those in the USA where bread is usually made out of flour enriched with artificial vitamins (to which I am personally allergic). One wonders what processing the flour has undergone that it needs these added synthetic vitamins, when they should have been there in the first place.

As far as possible, I eat organic food. Some raw food including meat is thought to protect against aging and degeneration. In England it is now possible to buy a wide range of good organic products and eat a healthy diet at home, however one may have to neglect these rules when eating out. I do try to stick to the rules as regards mechanically recovered meat on all occasions. Locally grown organic veggi-boxes are now available in many areas and can be delivered to the home, the quality is excellent, the foods sent will be seasonal and the varieties used will be much wider than those regularly appearing in supermarkets. The flavour is a whole new experience.

Farmers are beginning to realise that if they wish to have grandchildren, they will need to farm organically. Organic (or any) food loses its "life force" over time, and is of no value unless fresh. The best organic food is a gift of fresh, recently picked vegetables from a neighbour's pesticide free garden. Wash all non-organic salad to remove residues of chemicals used in growth and transport, and also "foggers" (sprays) used in some stores to keep insect pests at bay.

Washing will **not** remove the pesticides and fungicides actually incorporated in the plant during growth, from spraying as part of agriculture. I hear that many fruits and vegetables are sprayed up to 17 times, and with a variety of *different* pesticides. The testing of pesticides for safety is done singly, so the use of multiple chemicals in this way represents a massive experiment conducted on humankind.

Drinking water (and that used for soups and steaming vegetables) is best filtered, as there may be undesirable residues, although the authorities will deny this. In any case much drinking water has already been through four sets of kidneys. A good quality water filter is an asset. Alternatively good quality spring water can be purchased.

Bowel Health and the Immune System

The health of our intestinal flora (the bacterial population inside the bowel) is intimately bound up with the health of our immune system, and explains why people with candida and yeast problems in the gut tend to develop food and inhalant allergies. This is a nasty vicious circle and it deteriorates unless changes are made. Added to this, the unhealthy gut flora (bugs) produce a toxin (poison) as part of their life and death cycle, this is then absorbed into the sufferer's system, along with the food, causing depression, mood swings and a further load on the immune system.

Cynic's Corner

"The meek shall inherit the earth" ... but we can be sure that the multinationals are going to contest the will.

Chapter 4

Irritable Bowel Syndrome

Case History

Nora

A typical patient of mine with this problem was Nora. She was 48 years old when she came to see me with of a gradual onset, over five years, of weight gain, bloating and wind, water retention (ankle swelling,) joint pains, mood swings and feeling constantly tired. Dieting had failed to reduce her weight problem.

Nora had a responsible job in the armed services and was extremely capable. She had had a hysterectomy eight years before I met her and had suffered a difficult infection which had required several courses of antibiotics.

She lived in a semi-detached house with a garden near a river. She was a keen gardener and had noticed her symptoms were worse after mowing the grass, especially early in the season. She also had many indoor plants, which caused condensation on the insides of the windows.

When Nora first came to see me she had, at my request, been keeping a food diary, which included observations about the weather and how she felt on wet or damp days. This, together with a careful history, enabled me to diagnose a candida problem following her operation and courses of antibiotics.

Nora embarked on a basic anti-candida diet avoiding sugar, yeast, most cheeses, anything fermented, wilted or visibly mouldy, and increasing her intake of olive oil and garlic. I suggested nutritional supplements, including probiotics, which replace the intestinal "good bugs" originally killed by the antibiotic She felt worse during the first week due to a die-off reaction, from the anti-candida effect, but was aware that this was a good sign and persevered.

Perhaps the most important part of her treatment was reducing the total load of mould in her life. This involved getting rid of house-plants, drying the air with a dehumidifier and making liberal use of central heating. I also suggested that she use low light heating in damp corners, have any obvious mould removed (by someone else) and avoid cutting the grass.

Gradually Nora improved on this regime. After some weeks, she was able to broaden her diet. As her morning diarrhoea was cured, she was delighted to find that she could attend camp. Her mood and energy had returned to normal, her joints were better and she had lost some weight.

She still felt depressed in damp weather but was able to cope now that she understood why and could tighten up on the anti-candida diet at times when her symptoms threatened to return.

Most of the information in this chapter also applies to people with chronic food and inhalant allergies (mould, pollens, dust and house dust mites). I suspect most cases of IBS diagnosed by conventional doctors are really a combination of candida overgrowth and allergy, by another name. This book does not address acute (Type A) food allergies, often to nuts, which are life-threatening emergencies and require urgent medical treatment to avoid fatality. Complete avoidance of the allergen (food) concerned is mandatory.

IBS usually presents with bowel symptoms including diarrhoea and constipation, bloating worse towards evening, wind and much general discomfort. Added to this there may be any combination of the following:

General Symptoms
- Mood swings
- Depression
- Anxiety
- Obesity unresponsive to dietary restriction

Localised Symptoms
- Urinary problems, frequency, recurrent infections
- Joint pains
- Urgent diarrhoea, worst mornings
- Abdominal bloating, worsening as the day goes on
- Swelling of legs and ankles

Predisposing Factors and Events
- Several courses of antibiotics
- Steroid (hydrocortisone-like) drugs
- Stressful lifestyle
- History of child abuse
- Junk food diet
- Previous substance abuse
- Parasitic infestation

Women
- Use of birth control pills
- Fertility hormones (IVF)
- HRT
- Past history of a hysterectomy, especially complicated by infection and antibiotics.

These events may have occurred as much as five years before the IBS becomes obvious, but the change in intestinal bacteria causing gut

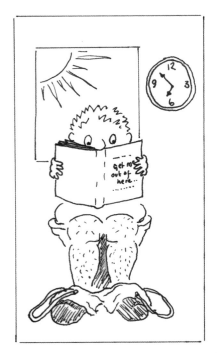
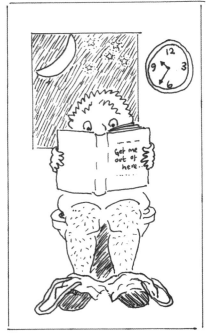

fermentation occurs gradually over a number of years. Palliatives from the chemist may have kept it in check for some time before it finally becomes unmanageable.

The diagnosis is straightforward if one is aware of the condition. A detailed history is helpful, but physical examination usually only confirms the site of pain and any complications, and adds little to the overall picture. Blood tests are often normal, and at present, specific testing for food allergies is unreliable, and may result in an unnecessarily restricted diet which does not address the true problem. Hopefully *accurate* tests for food allergy will eventually become available.

Blood tests are available in London (Biolab, appendix 2) for specific vitamin and mineral shortages, and poisonings with metals, and a thyroid function test should be part of this protocol, as poor thyroid function can complicate the picture. Stool tests for parasites should be done through the patient's own GP.

Before I see a patient, I ask them to make a food diary, which is a device to help *them* to learn to think environmentally about their life. This is a list of food and drink consumed at each meal, and should include the weather (as an indication of the mould count) and severity of any specific symptoms that vary, and/or how well they felt (energy level). They should also bring to the consultation any food supplements, vitamins and other medication they are taking. All this will assist with accurate diagnosis. Most cases of IBS respond to the following dietary and household changes, which I call my "Toolkit", and is extracted from the information sheet given to patients at their consultation.

Dietary Information for Allergy, Candida Problems and IBS

Be good to yourself, these are guidelines, not guilt-trips. A very noticeable improvement in symptoms and energy usually occurs after about six weeks of following this regime.

The aim is to reduce the numbers of moulds, yeasts and candida organisms in the gut, by starving them of sugar, their favorite nutrient, and replacing them with a supplement of acidophilus bacteria which are helpful. Foods to be avoided are those which encourage yeast growth. They include other yeasts, (cheese, alcohol and yeasted bread) and fruit which contains sugar. Carbohydrates, which can be converted easily into sugars during digestion, should be eaten only in limited amounts at the beginning.

Novel foods such as Quorn and Tofu are the result of fermentaton using a species of Aspergillus mould and are unsuitable for those with fungal and yeast related health problems. Soy sauce is also fermented.

Basic Anti Candida Diet: (for a few weeks until feeling better)

Avoid:
- Sugar (honey, syrup &c)
- Fruit other than apples, maximum two per day
- Yeast (use soda bread)
- Cheese except Gouda, Edam & cottage
- Alcohol, vinegar (use lemon juice in olive oil for salad dressing)
- Anything with visible mould on it and wilted green leaves
- (Mushrooms may be unhelpful at this stage.)

Do Eat:
- Extra virgin olive oil
- Raw garlic

(Both have anti Candida effects.)

Unlimited Quantities of:
- Meat
- Fish
- Vegetables and salads
- Eggs

Reasonable Quantities of Carbohydrates including:
- Brown rice
- Potatoes, buckwheat (related to the rhubarb food family, not to wheat)
- Pasta
- Millet
- Soda bread (un-yeasted bread), either home made or it can be bought at small bakeries (but check by inquiry that they really haven't added yeast).

The Hay Diet (food combining) helps people with energy loss, wind, bloating, candida, food allergies, weight problems and arthritis to feel better rapidly by reducing gut fermentation. It is described on page 26, and can be combined with the anti-candida diet to great benefit.

Some people will actually feel markedly worse after using this diet for a few days, this is a good sign and is caused by a "die off" (Herxheimer) reaction, because the dead candida and yeast organisms are liberating a toxin which is being absorbed into the body. It is unpleasant, but an indication to persevere with the diet, and be less active for a few days. It will improve spontaneously.

Food Supplements, Minerals and Vitamins

Use a yeast-free form of the following:
- Magnesium
- Selenium
- Zinc
- Multivitamin especially Vitamin B group
- Garlic
- Acidophilus
- Evening Primrose oil.

My approach to the treatment of IBS is similar to that for food and inhalant allergy, and there is probably a big overlap of pathology and causes. It may be true that the "label" a particular patient gets depends on the doctor he or she sees. There are always two sides to the coin, the things we eat and the contents of the air we breathe; and both need to be cleaned up for there to be a noticeable long-term improvement of symptoms.

Chronic Food Allergy

The symptoms are similar to IBS, and mood swings may be prominent. Rather like addiction (and possibly identical with it (chapter 12)) another dose of the offending food (the hair of the dog) will temporarily relieve the symptoms. The commonest culprit foods are wheat and dairy products, although other foods may be implicated and soya is becoming a problem. Chocolate is a common food causing allergy, and this also looks particularly like addiction ("Chocaholics").

Because food allergy is usually accompanied by candida overgrowth and a weakened immune system (from the toxic overload produced by the candida) measures to reduce the latter problem often result in a disappearance of the food allergies, without specific allergy treatment beyond a temporary removal of the offending food from the diet. Different therapists approach things differently, but I find that reduction of the "total load" by reducing the candida population and attendant toxicity, does cause a major improvement and return of tolerance for previously allergic foods. However if this does not occur, or the person has multiple major food allergies, then referral to a clinic specialising in Neutralisation (a type of Immunotherapy) p49 is helpful, and will enable the patient to eat a tolerable diet.

Confirming the Diagnosis

Currently, the available diagnostic tests are expensive and not particularly reliable in distinguishing allergic foods in individual patients, and I do not rely on them. I question the value of food allergy tests, since moulds are not tested for, all food has a mould component, and many people are mould sensitive. A food diary kept over 10 days will often reveal a great deal and most patients have a pretty good idea anyway. The easiest but not "scientifically provable" way is to omit suspect foods, one at a time for at least a week, and notice the effect of removal (withdrawal symptoms?) and subsequent improvement, and the effect of eating the food after a period of abstinence (which may cause a dramatic unpleasant reaction). A diet omitting dairy products or/and wheat is difficult to sustain unless one is prepared to cook everything from scratch, as wheat and casein from milk are added to most processed food.

The more medically favoured method (considered "scientific," although all of this, and life in general, is subjective) is to subsist for some days on the Caveman Diet (which consists largely of pears, lamb, sweet potatoes and some unspeakable margarine closely resembling axle grease, plus limited carbohydrates) to which no-one is supposed to be allergic, and then add in regular foods, one at a time every two or three days, noticing the effect. There are two problems with this. It is impossible to do and have a normal life (and sounds like a recipe for nutritional disaster). Also, since all foods have a mould content, the person may be having a reaction to the *moulds* in the food thereby confusing the issue.

Crank diets in which a number of major food groups are omitted, if sustained over a period of time will result in nutritional deficiencies as well as disruption to social life.

Chapter 5

Mould and other Inhalant Allergies

These are allergies to things breathed into the lungs from the air, including pollens, moulds, dust and house dust mite faeces. Multiple Chemical Sensitivity is described in chapter 8.

I have a fantasy that, one day we will have a machine that will allow us to see what air *looks* like. The nearest we have now is the horror shown up by a sunbeam at a certain angle, when all the dust is exposed to view. Dust is a mixture containing mould spores, pollens and general debris. To continue my fantasy with a mythological sample of outdoor air, we would find layers of some of the following substances, the heavier ones would be nearer the ground: a mist of moulds and dusts, pollens, some chemical pollutants, especially where these are sprayed frequently, water vapour, and particles of all kinds.

Indoor air would contain many of the outdoor pollutants and mould, but in a lesser concentration, together with any chemicals off-gassed by newish carpets and furnishings, a spectrum of indoor moulds, dust, cigarette residue and much else.

My fantasy includes a way of showing all these substances in a full colour representation of an air sample, it would be alarming, but could provide the impetus for change.

Pollen, Grass and Tree Allergies may produce asthma, hay fever or general symptoms. Conventional medical treatment brings relief by suppressing symptoms pharmaceutically, but does nothing to alleviate the cause. There are also techniques of immunotherapy which help the body overcome the problem. (Provocative Neutralisation and Enzyme Potentiated Desensitisation (EPD) see page 49.) If pollen allergy does not entirely fit the season of pollination (see chart appendix 3) of the suspect plant, one should consider mould allergy as part of the problem and try the precautions mentioned below.

House Dust Mites

Many people are allergic to the *faeces* of these mites that invisibly infest our beds and pillows. They are breathed in during the night and produce a range of allergic symptoms including asthma. Environmental control of the bed and surrounding area can reduce this (see section below under moulds). Specific desensitisation as mentioned for pollens may help considerably.

Mould Allergy

Moulds are everywhere in the air, and there are several thousand different species. They are visible on vegetables and on the inside walls of some houses, where they appear as black areas or dots. Houses with much visible mould should be avoided when purchasing as de-moulding houses is very difficult.

While there may be no obvious visible mould, many people are allergic to the moulds in the air they breathe. Moulds are very small particles in the air, (0.3 microns) and together with dust and other items, they are impossible to filter out as they pass through the filters and redistribute themselves unless the latter are constantly cleaned.

Currently we have no instrument to measure mould count in air; a meter or electronic counter would be immensely useful. We also have no way of instantly distinguishing which mould affects people or houses, nor whether it is the mould, or a toxin produced by it, which causes the problem. The best available measurements are done through exposing agar (jelly) culture medium plates in the rooms concerned, and having a public analyst's laboratory culture and identify the moulds, which takes several weeks and is quite costly.

The Symptoms of Mould Allergy

Many of the symptoms are identical with those of IBS and sometimes, food allergy, probably because moulds are part of the cause in these conditions, however the following are more marked in mould allergy:

- Gross mood swings including depression (paralysing in the mornings)
- Acute fear and panic with rapid heart (often treated by cardiologists with anticoagulants and cardioversion) this is usually worse at 3am and involves waking up terrified night after night, and may eventually develop into fear of going to sleep.
- Bouts of energy loss to the point of total inertia, where the thought of doing anything at all is quite impossible.
- Joint pains usually leading to arthritis in large weight-bearing joints.

These symptoms may vary in intensity depending on the weather. They may also be much worse in some houses than others.

Other General Symptoms
- Obesity unresponsive to dietary restriction
- Symptoms as under IBS (page 35)

Localised Symptoms
- "Hay Fever" and nasal symptoms
- Asthma
- Urinary problems, frequency
- Joint pains
- Flatulence, abdominal bloating
- Swelling of legs and ankles

A mould allergy sufferer may notice major changes in the way they feel and the bits that hurt when the weather changes for the worse, and be much better in hot *dry* climates. When it rains, the mould count rises with the damp, when there is a gale blowing, the moulds involved in decomposing vegetable matter are thrown into the air. There is a massive increase in the mould count before a thunder storm (which may sour milk and make swimming pools turn green). This may account for the huge rise in deaths and hospital admissions from childhood asthma now being seen. Sadly my consultant colleagues are largely unaware of mould allergy, probably because we can not see or count moulds, as yet.

As many of the specific symptoms of mould allergy could be construed as psychiatric or cardiological (heart related) it is easy to see how people may get referred to the wrong medical department and wind up on tranquilisers or heart drugs. There are very few specialist allergy clinics, and almost all of them are run privately, and not as part of the NHS.

A pollen allergy which extends outside the specific pollen season is usually really a mould allergy. Also there is a tie-up with candida and yeast overgrowth problems in the intestines, and each will make the other worse, as all three organisms are from the mould family (Fungi).

As a long term sufferer from mould allergy (for which there are no specific tests) I have, by subjective observation and personal research, become an expert on the environmental aspects of this problem. One of the more distressing symptoms is acute terror in mouldy houses and worst in the night, almost suggesting a haunting until one works out the real cause. I suspect many people with intermittent panic attacks and morning depression may have a missed diagnosis of mould allergy. The symptoms improve dramatically after a few hours away from the mouldy house, only to recur shortly after returning to the source of the problem, when the moulds are again inhaled through the lungs, which are a very efficient entry point into the body.

Unless causing specific problems such as asthma, mould allergy is difficult to treat with conventional drugs, however some of the recent antihistamines are well worth a try. I find that Periactin, available over the counter in the UK, is some help. People will vary. Claritin (another over the counter medication) may also work to a limited extent.

Caveat: *Do not combine Antihistamines with Immunotherapy, the combination will make you very much worse.*

Emergency Action to Abort an Attack of Mould Allergy/ Candida

1. Don't eat (temporarily) this reduces "total load." Drink water, some people find tea helps.
2. Take an anti-Candida preparation or drug if possible, for a short time.
3. Take pepto-bismol tablets 2 four times daily with medicinal charcoal.
4. Remember all this is only temporary, and will go away. You are *not* going permanently mad.
5. Use of Nasal Airguard may help (from "Healthy House").
6. Restart food gradually using anti-Candida diet and food combining.
7. *Fix the house.*

Immunotherapy see p49 will help but is not the whole answer, and should be combined with the anti-candida diet (which can be relaxed in good climates) and environmental control of airborne moulds.

Diagnosis of Mould Allergy is usually by elimination, and should be considered in those with food and other allergies that do not respond completely to immunotherapy for the food items suspected. If neutralisation therapy using mould mixes reduces or abolishes the symptoms, then the diagnosis is made. Since this is by default, and many doctors are unaware of the problem, mould allergy is very often missed. I make a point of listening to what *the patient suspects*, which is often correct.

Nobody knows their body better than its owner, despite the old paternalistic attitude that "doctor knows best".

Environmental Control of Mould Allergy

The mould count in the air we breathe varies directly with the ambient humidity level. A cheap humidity meter which also measures temperature, is a huge help. Since England has a humid climate, the ambient humidity in a house may be about 60% or more, and mould will be present in the air. Having a cold climate, it is simple to reduce the internal humidity by central heating and dehumidifiers (air driers.) The latter should be run constantly, with plumbed outlets, allowing the water they extract to be drained outside. Even with best intentions, people will forget to empty the water reservoir on a long-term basis, and it will fill up and need emptying daily. Dehumidifiers stop working when the reservoir is full. To have any effect, they need to be run on maximum setting in perpetuity. The aim is to reduce the ambient humidity to around 35 – 40%, which some people will find too dry. This keeps the moulds out of the air and is particularly important for bedrooms. It is worth keeping one room mould free and using this for most purposes, if possible.

Kitchens and bathrooms are inherently damp, vent fans should be used. Never dry clothes on radiators. Only open windows when the weather is dry and close them at dusk, the night air is humid. One is trying to create a dry "micro-climate" in, at least, part of the house. Ventilate cupboards. Use Dimplex style low light space heaters in damp, cold corners. Have central heating come on early in the morning, many moulds "sporulate" (reproduce in huge numbers) in the night and early morning.

An Air Purifier (p129) of the type that generates ozone (not harmful and very cleansing) may help considerably. Like all fans and filters (including those in dehumidifiers) it will need cleaning monthly or it will clog with dust and then stop functioning effectively.

Airfree (p129) This ingenious gadget removes dust and mould from the air by heat (without itself getting particularly hot) and requires no filters or cleaning. It takes four weeks for the full effect to occur, and must be left on constantly in a particular room (and not moved from room to room). It is certainly effective, since using one in my kitchen the Basil plants stopped getting mould, and started to thrive instead of suffering a lingering death. The average house would require at least two Airfrees, one in the bedroom and one elsewhere, perhaps in the kitchen.

Air Conditioning

Air Conditioners can be mould traps which distribute mould spores round the house. The plant and ducts should be regularly cleaned by professionals and the filter changed or cleaned monthly. Ideally an ultra-violet lamp can be installed near the air inlet to the plant, this should remove moulds from the air prior to cooling and circulation. Inlet vents in the floor are a bad idea as they circulate dust and mould from the floor and carpet. More modern systems with the vents in the ceiling are much better.

Air conditioners can often be greatly improved by running an ozone generating electric air freshener through the air outlet vent (large square grill which leads to the exterior fan and air-conditioning machinery) while the system is set on "recycle." It will have the effect of killing the moulds in the ventilation shafts and plant. This can be done for several hours while one is out, with the ozone generator on maximum, and then turned off or low, on ones return.

The "dangers" of breathing ozone are tightly bound with the nitric acid and other pollutants in traffic-fume laden air, breathing ozone made by these generators does not cause problems in sensible dilutions of room air and contains none of the other harmful pollutants.

House Furnishings

These comments also apply to house dust mite (faeces) allergy. Since old carpets and bedding eventually grow mould and harbour house dust mites (HDMs) an ideal house would have stone floors and washable rugs, but one may get away with modern, largely synthetic carpets.

Beds as for carpets, bedding and mattresses harbour mould and HDMs. All mattresses will eventually get mould, so one solution is a waterbed, which is plastic, and minimal bedclothes which can be washed. To prevent HDMs and moulds, it is worth doing the following to duvets and blankets prior to washing, in order to remove particulate matter:

Put the duvet in a large black bin liner, put the sucker end of the vacuum cleaner tube *without carpet attachment* into the bag with the duvet, connect the other end to the vacuum cleaner and switch on, wrapping the plastic bag around sucker pipe so that the cleaner sucks out all the air (and dust etc.) and the duvet is reduced to a small proportion of original size (see diagram opposite). Turn off the cleaner and allow air to enter the plastic bag. Next launder the duvet. (Cold water washes do *not* kill HDMs.)

1. Tube of vacuum cleaner (no atachment) goes into black bin liner – hold ends of bin liner –

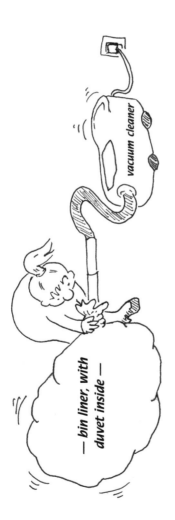

— bin liner, with duvet inside —

vacuum cleaner

2. — sucks all air, moulds and mites into vaccuum — duvet shrinks to a tiny package.

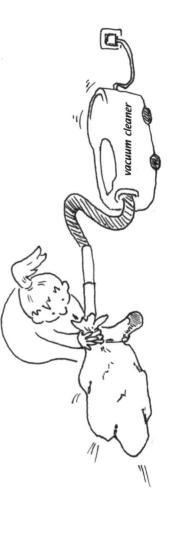

vacuum cleaner

This procedure can also be used for pillows. Pillows and mattresses should be encased in non-porous zipped covers, which keep the moulds and HDMs from the user's nose. Buy cheap synthetic pillows, they may be laundered once before going lumpy, then replace. Wash the outer pillow case frequently, the nose is in intimate contact with the pillow.

When staying in hotels it is worth taking a synthetic pillow and spreading a black bin-liner (opened out) below the bottom sheet, over the head and chest area of the bed, to distance oneself from what may be a very dusty/mouldy mattress. It is a good idea to remove the bin liner next day, lest the chamber-maid thinks one suffers from an unusual form of incontinence.

In spite of all these precautions the mould count will vary, and sufferers may feel worse in wet weather, high wind and, particularly just before a thunder storm. In general simple facial masks do not help as mould particles are so small (0.3microns) that they go through the material. An industrial gasmask of the type used to protect workmen against spray paint and chemicals (available from hardware stores in USA) would work, but are not practical on a long term basis. They can be used for dusty jobs.

Nasal Airguard (from the makers www.nasalairguard.com or the Healthy House p129) is a recent invention designed to prevent pollen allergy, it should also help with mould allergy and consists of two small filters joined by a plastic link. One filter goes up each nostril and they last up to 24 hours. I find them quite effective and certainly worth taking when staying away from home.

Plants and Gardens

Unfortunately the garden is a hotbed of moulds, and most jobs stir them up so that they are inhaled by the gardener. Those with mould allergy should avoid mowing grass (or being outside near anyone else mowing grass) which, particularly at the first cut in March/April, throws up a huge mould load into the air; a similar effect is produced on farms by harvesting and hay/silage cutting in the summer. Avoid working with compost, dying foliage etc. I find it wisest to avoid gardening altogether. It is sensible not to have house plants, but confine oneself to artificial floral arrangements indoors. Conservatories with plants are not helpful as they encourage moisture and moulds which tend to get into the rest of the house. Any windows running with condensation in the mornings are an indication of damp air in the house.

The use of garden sprinklers throws up a mist of mould-laden droplets which one will breathe, and which will cause symptoms. Presumably the intervals between use allow moulds to grow in the stagnant water in the hose or piping, ready to be ejected as an aerosol on next usage. One can hold ones breath when passing these, but one should avoid standing nearby, especially when they first come on.

Immunotherapy (Known as "allergy shots")

There are currently two forms of Immunotherapy available for treating food and inhalant allergies, and either may produce a remarkable improvement in symptoms, although, in my view, neither provides the complete answer to mould allergy, probably because we are not yet able to identify all the moulds which cause allergies, or because part of the problem is a temporary toxic poisoning from the moulds, rather than an allergic reaction.

The mechanism by which these treatments work is not fully understood, but they seem to increase the immune system's tolerance to the allergen concerned and make the patient feel very much better.

Both methods of immunotherapy are time consuming in different ways, and neither is widely available on the NHS.

Provocative Neutralisation

Each suspected allergic item (food or inhalant) is tested separately by small injection into the upper arm, and the end point (the dilution of the allergen which turns off the allergic reaction and its symptoms) is found and noted. This process is repeated for each suspected allergen, and a bottle is made up containing the "neutralising dose" of each allergen tested. This is then used by the patient at home, injecting a measured small dose into the thigh muscle on alternate days. The intervals are gradually increased until the treatment is no longer needed.

For some this works admirably, and although the testing is time consuming, the experience of listening to the more experienced patients in the testing room is most educational for the "beginner". The main problem is spontaneous change in the neutralising end point, so that retesting is needed.

Neutralisation with Dilutions of 'Flu Vaccine for Virus Infections

This approach can be used to turn off the symptoms of virus infections including 'flu, herpes simplex and zoster, glandular fever and possibly other viruses illnesses, but not, unfortunately, the common cold.

The person should visit the allergy clinic when well and be tested. They will receive a bottle each of 'flu vaccine at a two and three times dilution, which is kept in the frig. at home, until needed. At the onset of 'flu the "three" dilution strength (weaker) is usually needed first, and will stop the symptoms dramatically. Injections may be needed every half-hour initially, but the intervals can be lengthened, and a point will be reached when the *stronger* number two dilution will work better. Vast sums and many lives could be saved if this procedure was available on the NHS (which is probably why it is not).

Some people with mould allergy feel better if they have a regular injection of 'flu vaccine (probably on the number two dilution, but trial and error is needed, as the end-point can vary). Presumably allergy to viruses is part of the "total load" in some people.

Enzyme Potentiated Desensitisation (EPD)

This is a single injection of a wide range of allergens including food, moulds and chemicals, combined with an enzyme which makes it work. It is given at intervals of at least three months, and may allow the body to build up resistance, over time, to the allergens concerned. The intervals can be extended and the injections eventually discontinued.

The down side to EPD is the preparation for each dose. In order to make the enzyme/allergen system work, the patient must avoid all allergic foods for one week before and about two weeks after the injection, and for the three days surrounding the injection day must stick to an extremely restricted and unpleasant diet and try to keep away from inhalants such as mould. It may also be necessary to take an anti-fungal drug for the week prior to the injection. All of this makes it necessary to plan ahead for an EPD dose by keeping the week concerned free of social functions involving food. It does work well, but in my experience the dose may not last the full three months and one should not have them more frequently.

Some people will try both methods (at different times) especially if one method did not succeed.

Chapter 6

More about Moulds

Some people will realise, after reading the previous chapter and using some of the suggestions, that they really are allergic to moulds, and that while the dietary changes help over a bad patch, these are not the whole solution. This chapter is for them, and goes more deeply into the life of moulds and fungi, and what to avoid. Much of this has been learned through my own observations as a mould allergy sufferer. I have not found any books on moulds as they affect human health, though there is a variety of useful publications on the Internet, under headings of moulds (spelt molds in the USA) and building practices for improving houses. I have not so far located any expert on moulds and fungi who has related their knowledge to human health, and so decided to become expert myself, by learning and observation.

Houses

Obviously it is vital to ensure that water does not come into the house and to fix leaks very quickly. Condensation is a problem in kitchens and bathrooms, and needs extractor fans. A temperature gradient where there is cold air outside and warm air inside may cause condensation, a builder should be able to fix this. Undoubtedly drying the air by dehumidification will help mould allergics to feel better at home.

I suspect it takes three or more years of living (unknowingly) in an invisibly mouldy house for the symptoms to start. As these are usually related to tiredness, energy loss, depression anxiety and fear or terror in the night, the diagnosis is often missed by the sufferer and the doctor. Tranquilisers do not help and carry a long-term risk of addiction.

Geopathic Stress and "Total Load"

Geopathic stress (Chapter 7) causes some houses to have a bad energetic feel and often leads to allergy and other ill health. Where someone is suffering from mould allergy, this should always be investigated by a competent dowser (on site, or using a map of the house and surroundings) and the draining energies should be corrected. Living in a house with Geopathic stress will make it very difficult to treat mould allergy, as the former massively adds to "total load" and may even encourage mould growth. In this modern electromagnetic era it is worth considering electrical sensitivity as a component of "total load" and the proximity of houses to mobile phone and TETRA masts. The Neutralec disc (see below) should help considerably with this and with geopathic stress. Leaving mobile phones switched on and their frequent use, other than for occasional emergencies, is probably a bad idea.

Furnishings

Beds and pillows are a big problem, do the symptoms come on when one goes to bed? If so consider that the bed, mattress or pillows may be mouldy and replace them. Enclosing mattresses and pillows in non-porous covers may help, but as mould spores are so small, these covers must be waterproof and will not "breathe", which creates heat and perspiration problems. Is the carpet old? If so remove it and consider bare floors around the bed. Beds are nearer the floor than our noses are when we are up and about, I have always suspected that this may contribute to mould symptoms occurring mainly at night. Would the upper bunk be better? I have not tried this.

Biology of Moulds

Fungi is the family name for the following:
- Moulds
- Yeasts
- Candida sp.
- Mushrooms including toadstools and much else.

All fungi multiply by means of spores which settle on suitable surfaces and send out an invisible network of filaments called a mycellium which spreads through the material and draws nourishment from it. The spores are very small particles and there may be millions of them in the air.

Where?
Moulds are everywhere and they can cause allergic and toxic reactions.

We inhale them or eat them in food, they require moisture and prefer dark unventilated places. Those studies that have been done in an effort to measure mould count and identify which moulds grow inside houses and outside in the corresponding gardens, suggest that inside mould species are a reflection of outside moulds, but in smaller numbers.

My own observation is that if I am forced to stay inside my house for a few days (a cold, perhaps) my arthritis gets better, only to recur when I start going outside. The reason could be related to the lack of exercise or some strange effect of the virus that kept me in, but I suspect is really the lack of exposure to the outside moulds which contribute to arthritis in some people, especially those people whose pain is much worse in damp weather.

Appearance

Moulds are the black dots you see on damp walls, or white mildew visible on food, walls, shoes etc. Mostly they are invisible. You can smell their presence in damp houses.

When

Moulds sporulate (breed) all the year round, but the highest airborne levels are in July and August (harvest time) there is another peak in April when the massed ranks of suburban lawn mowers make their first cut, as the grass has stood all winter allowing mould growth and the moulds are then thrown into the air. The autumnal leaf rotting season causes another peak.

Common moulds which can cause allergies:
- Alternaria Tenuis
- Aspergillus sp.
- Penicillium sp.
- Cladosporium Herbarum
- Candida Albicans

and many more.

Outside moulds and fungi may make a massive invisible network of mycelium which extends underground. It is worth watching what grows in the garden, including little brown toadstools in the autumn which I regard as a sign of high outside mould count. The Fungi family includes moulds, mushrooms and toadstools and some people will probably be allergic to the airborne spores of toadstools. Many of these have elaborate triggering mechanisms to liberate billions of spores into the air (puffballs are an example). High winds distribute spores effectively into the air and cause a high count, as does the muggy humid weather just before a thunder storm. In both situations I can notice the changes physically.

I do not know of any research on this, but I am able to eat ordinary and Portobello mushrooms without problems, but Cep mushrooms are a disaster. Those who are mould allergic should probably view the up-market fungi and unusual mushrooms now available in supermarkets, with some suspicion. There are now some alternative wonder cures which are made from Japanese and other fungi, and the same comment applies.

Algae are closely related to moulds. I find that blue green algae, so touted for their health benefits, have made me ill for days. Also vitamin B is usually of yeast or fermented origin, and causes me appalling side effects. Quorn, Tofu and Soy Sauce are fermented from species of Aspergillus moulds in industrial sized vats, one can assume that fragments of the moulds will remain in the food after the fermentation and any filtration process.

The problem of novel and fermented foods will get worse as the food industry is using Aspergillus mould in more applications, without realising that it is a common allergen, and species of Fusarium mould are being used in the complicated process of genetic modification of food, especially in the USA. My observation that mould is a much greater health problem in houses in the USA may be related to this, or to other factors.

Antibiotics

Many antibiotics (penicillin is the classic) are made from moulds, my experience is that I am not allergic to these, the only problem being the tendency of all antibiotics to kill off the beneficial lactobacilli in the intestine leading to candida overgrowth, which then makes mould allergy worse later. (See Chapter 4 for the remedy for this.)

Outdoors

Avoid garden sprinklers, proximity to grass being (or having recently been) mowed, compost, greenhouses, etc. The mould count is higher in high winds and Autumn, also April (grass cutting) and August (harvest) and just before a thunderstorm. Some people think that a good rain shower washes the moulds out of the air, others (including me) think that rain encourages mould growth and therefore raises the airborne count.

Someone has observed that in general the mould count rises around dawn or sunrise, and also near dusk or sunset. Certainly using the timer to start the central heating around 6.00 am helps considerably in the winter by drying the air. If one gets a bad mould attack in late August, after not having the heating on for some months, this may be because mould and humidity gradually build up in the house, and choosing a cool day to run the heating for a few hours (with some ventilation) will produce a dramatic improvement. Unfortunately running heating and dehumidifiers is expensive. It is, however, cheaper and safer than doctors and pills, and for a self-employed person, will increase energy, work output and quality of life out of all proportion to the expense.

Food

Revert temporarily to the basic anti-candida diet (avoiding sugar and anything fermented or mouldy). Refer back to chapter 5. Avoid food with visible mould or wilted; anything made from mould (Quorn and other myco-proteins, soy sauce etc.); most cheese (ripe cheeses owe their delights to moulds). Remember the "Total Load Effect" of a meal.

General Health Measures

Many mould allergy sufferers are deficient in vitamins (especially the B group) and minerals. If there is no major improvement after taking a good vitamin and mineral supplement for a few weeks (preferably in liquid form to aid its intake into the body from the intestine, pills may go unchanged down the loo) then tests should be done.

Biolab (p127) do tests to identify mineral and vitamin shortages (and much else,) and which can then be put right. These investigations must be arranged through a doctor who can interpret and advise on the results.

Full Spectrum Lightboxes in the Winter

Since "mould folk" often feel worst in the mornings and getting up can be devastating; it seems logical to consider a Lightbox (see under SAD, chapter 16) I am not aware that this has been tried before, so it is something of a shot in the dark.

Ozone Generating Air Purifiers

These really do help keep bedroom air mould free. I use one set to come on when I am out at a low ozone level, for 2-3 hours, perhaps twice weekly once the situation has stabilised. Air purifiers should be located as high up as possible and the filter changed or cleaned monthly.

Air Filters and Ionisers

Air filters clog up with dust and mould and redistribute the latter throughout the room. I have not found them useful, their air currents tend to stir things up which are better left undisturbed. For me ionisers make no noticeable difference. Some people find they help, they certainly collect dust.

Airfree (p129)

As mentioned in chapter 5 these are worth having and will keep a bedroom mould free. They have no filters and require no maintenance.

Neutralec Personal Protection Discs (p129)

These have protective frequencies incorporated into the plastic from which they are made, and somehow block the body's allergic reaction. (I do not know the detailed mechanism for this.) These discs have made a huge difference to my health and the inconveniences and difficulties of a "bad mould day" but this is an entirely subjective comment. I have tried other pendent gadgets for improving energy or blocking computer and mobile phone emanations, none of which really worked for me, but we are all different.

Finally…

Become your own detective, start noticing what preceeded a bad reaction (cold shakes, sudden energy loss etc.) what did you just breathe, where were you? What food or made up dish have you recently eaten? Study the ingredient list if from a supermarket. What did you eat or did you use a new health supplement product *yesterday?* Some things have slow effects. All this is much easier when one doesn't have bad days every day, making it easier to spot the ups and downs.

It is helpful to keep a diary or note the dates on which you had a bad attack, their seasonality becomes apparent after a year or two and confirms that the diagnosis is correct.

One really has to become ones own consultant at this; hospitals and most conventionally trained doctors are blissfully unaware of the mould connection to many illnesses. As mould is invisible and unprovable, one could be considered slightly mad or paranoid, and this does not help.

Be Optimistic, Mould Allergy can be Overcome …

Chapter 7

Houses, Hauntings, Underground Water and Electricity

There is a body of fascinating work from Germany and Scandinavia on "Cancer Houses" which describes how, when the crossings of under-ground streams (at different depths) occurred under someones bed, the occupants very frequently got cancer. This work was done in the 1930's by very competent water dowsers and the statistical correlation is startling. It was carried out in rural areas, where farmhouses were passed down the family, often with the marital bed staying in the same position for generations, with dire results.

More recent work by the late Wing Commander Beadon, a widely respected dowser, showed how underground water crossings adversely affected the health of a number of people living in a Surrey village. The map of underground water courses correlated convincingly with sick or troubled households.

In my own life and work experience I have found underground streams a very important aspect of the "energetic feel" of houses, and where the energies are unfavourable, improvements can be made.

Geopathic Stress is the term given to the draining energy field which occurs in some houses. Allergies and ill-health may result from the "energy drain" lowering the immune system. Other causes include unfavourable ley-lines (lines of force related to ancient monuments such as Stonehenge and standing stones). Magnetic flux, the break-up of the various earth energy grids, and Radon gas in some areas may also contribute to a draining energy in some houses. From the practical point of view, I confine my efforts to dealing with underground streams and their energies, which seems to cure the problem.

Each house and its occupants are individual and those affected will need to co-operate with a competent map, or on-site, dowser. (The British Society of Dowsers keeps a list. Appendix 2.) There are various ways of dealing with this, but I favour using a strategically placed metal stake, "up-stream" from the house, in the (dowsed) centre of the stream(s), done with respect for the earth and non-denominational prayer. If correctly placed, this approach results in a remarkable improvement which may be noticed in about 20 minutes by those sensitive to earth energies. (If the stake is inadvertently placed "downstream" from the house, it will make the situation very much worse.)

I strongly suspect there is a relationship between "black streams" (unfavourable underground water/energy) and the mould count in the air in some houses. One can not prove this, but it does seem logical to assume that an underground stream which does not flow freely may hold stagnant water, and that undesirable effects from this can be transmitted to the house above, either as dampness, mould or in some other not yet understood way.

Hauntings

There is an association between unfavourable earth energies and hauntings, I have experienced this when an unsuccessful attempt was made to change the energies in a house. The problem can be eliminated by correcting the geopathic stress affecting the house using the method outlined above, which could be described as a non-denominational exorcism. The British Society of Dowsers has information on the whole subject and can recommend dowsers who specialise in working with houses, either on site or by dowsing a plan of the house and garden, sent by mail or fax. (A donation should be included, dowsers usually do not charge fees.)

It may take several attempts to fix a house, and different dowsers may find different energies (and all may be correct). More than one stream may be causing trouble, this is likely if the problem keeps recurring, despite staking the stream. Earth energies may change or move over a period of time, so, if symptoms recur, it is worth having the site re-dowsed and altering the position of the stake accordingly.

Some dowsers prefer to remove the stake (seeing the operation as "earth acupuncture"). My experience was that the symptoms all came back when the stake was removed, and normality was achieved by leaving the stake in the earth, *but marked with an inverted plastic milk bottle and sign saying "do not remove."* It is worth joining ones local dowsing group and learning the technique (the BSD has phone numbers) the more experienced members will be delighted to help.

Electrical Phenomena Adversely Affecting Houses

Some people are very sensitive to various electrical phenomena, and suffer ill-health when living near electrical transformers, power lines or mobile phone masts. There are reports of chronically ill children whose health improved dramatically when their bed was moved away from the house "consumer unit" (incoming electrical main and associated fuse boxes and meters). Perhaps these people are analogous to those suffering from Multiple Chemical Sensitivity (chapter 8) and are the electrical version of the canary in the coal mine, something of an early warning to us all, at a time when we are increasingly surrounded by an invisible "smog" of electro-magnetic phenomena.

Houses

External Considerations

I would not buy a house situated near power lines, electrical transformers or mobile phone masts, however these may be added after one has purchased, and there are some things that one can do to mitigate harmful electrical effects.

Inside the House

The house wiring is accomplished in the form if a ring-main so that the wires go round the house and the current surrounds us. This may not be good for health. There is an increasing use of small, low voltage transformers powering individual items such as phones, computers and hi-fi. These transformers have been found to affect the lie of the pile of carpets, so one wonders what it is doing to us. It is worth trying to avoid sleeping or sitting for long periods in places that are near the following:

- House consumer unit
- Transformers
- Electric bed heaters and blankets (these should be *unplugged* from the mains at night.)
- Any rechargeable item, such as a telephone on its charger.
- Mobile phone or house cordless phone, unless switched *off*.

House Cordless Phones

These fall into two types, analogue, and the more recent digital phones. The latter can be shown with a meter to put out a high frequency electro-magnetic field over a wide area from the charger, and the handset output has the capability to affect the brain. These are best replaced by the older analogue type, whose electromagnetic field output is much less. A hard-wired phone on a long cord with a loud-speaker facility is much safer, as we do not know the long-term effects of exposing our brains to microwaves at close quarters.

Cellular Phones

Handsets

The above comments also apply to cell phones. The use of cell phones in cars is very unwise, because the metal body of the car allows the microwaves from the phone to rebound and "echo" multiplying the effect. If this information was made public, nobody would use their mobile phone in a car (moving or stationary) and the road safety aspects would not be an issue.

Cellular Phone Masts

There are two kinds, regular cellular phone masts (including 3G coming soon) and TETRA masts. There is much anecdotal evidence to suggest that there is an increase in cancer, leukaemias and other ill health in those living near mobile phone masts. Microwave measuring equipment (which can be hired from Healthy House p129) shows a huge increase in emanations near these masts (but not directly underneath, which is in the "lea"). Kinesiological (muscle strength) testing shows the weakening effects of this radiation on the body (and the protective effects of Nutralec Personal Protection Discs, p129).

TETRA masts are a new issue. TErrestrial Trunked RAdio is being foisted onto the police and emergency services to replace their existing radio frequency, which has been expensively sold by the government to the mobile phone companies. It has all the radiation problems of mobile phones and its data transmitting system pulses at a frequency of 17 cycles per second (cps). This will undoubtedly disrupt brain function in equipment users and those living near the masts, as it is our brain waves' beta frequency. (See Appendix 4 for full details of the mechanism.)

Despite strong local opposition, a major phone company is putting up these masts (in some cases without planning permission) on schools and hospitals as well as near homes. The masts have to be "line of sight" to work, so there will be a lot of them. Added to this, Railtrack is using the same system, and doesn't even need planning permission to put masts on their land, often outside peoples' homes.

The company concerned denies that the masts or handsets cause illness, using the old cry of the big battalions: "there is no evidence that our little marvel causes ill health." Have they done tests, if so how? In any case you can not prove a thing *doesn't* happen, only that it does.

Case Histories:

1. A *farmer allowed a mobile phone mast to be sited on his land twelve years ago. He has developed cancer, his son has moved away because of it and eight of his neighbours, in a small community, have also developed cancer. The farmer can not get out of the contract which still has a further eight years to run, and is desperate.*

2. *A cluster of leukaemia cases has occurred in a fishing village near Fife, Scotland, in the 12 years since a Dolphin mast (similar to TETRA) was installed nearby. This had previously been a very fit community.*

3. *A couple on the Isle of Wight became ill very soon after a TETRA mast sited close to their house "went live". They felt so ill that they could only use the basement of their house. They tried covering the windows with aluminium cooking foil, not only did this not help, but the foil developed unexplained holes with in a few days.*

The Powerwatch website (www.powerwatch.org.uk) has much more information on this whole subject and links to local groups trying to keep their back-yard TETRA-free, (which sadly, is a bit like farting against the thunder.)

Neutralec Personal Protection Discs (p129) are a newly developed product, a plastic disc is processed to incorporate protective frequencies against electromagnetic and other harmful phenomena, and they are extremely effective. The company also markets a plug-in neutraliser to deal with house electrical problems.

Chapter 8

Multiple Chemical Sensitivity (MCS) and Gulf War Syndrome

Thanks to the enormous increase in the production and use of synthetic chemicals in the last half century, we are now seeing people suffering from the results of chemical exposures, and for a variety of reasons, the diagnosis is being missed by doctors and discouraged by governments.

Case History

Janine was a 29-year-old salesperson for a cosmetics company and had done very well, achieving awards for her salesmanship. Her life was going well and the only notable past event was her childhood, which was affected by her father's alcoholism with constant rowing and arguments. Janine had to watch in impotent rage as her father regularly beat up her younger brother. She felt terrible anger and guilt that she could not intervene, and had learned to "stuff her feelings" in the interests of avoiding worse horrors.

One year after her office had been re-decorated, re-carpeted and had new air conditioning installed, she developed 'flu like symptoms, tiredness, exhaustion, depression and eventually found she could not work. Her GP was helpful but ignorant of Environmental Medicine, and suggested vitamins and time off. Much later Janine saw a magazine article by a doctor who was versed in MCS and arranged to consult her. Janine was advised to use the general measures suggested at the end of this chapter, and made a slow but steady recovery. She remained sensitive to the vapours out-gassed from carpets and Formica, and modified her house in order to work from home.

The best known group of sufferers from this condition come under the heading of "Gulf War Syndrome" and having spoken to sufferers, they are very badly disabled by it. These soldiers were given a cocktail of immunising injections at too short an interval before departure, and later were exposed to an unknown cocktail of chemicals including pesticides, vapours from burning oil wells, insecticides and possibly organophosphate nerve-gas used in chemical warfare.

Farmers and those who used sheep and cattle dip (organo-phosphates) and many other chemical workers are developing this problem after long term exposure.

Some of those who drank the water after the Camelford, Devon contamination incident have also developed this syndrome. Most people who develop MCS have no known cause, and one must assume that they are like the canary in the coal mine, something of a warning to the rest of us that there is a problem that we are neglecting to see. These people are a fast growing minority.

It is usually exposure to chemical *cocktails* that triggers the sensitivity in the first place. When commercial chemicals are tested for toxicity, single chemicals are used on laboratory animals in the short term, the effect of *combinations of chemicals* is not tested, neither is *the long term effect of chronic low dose exposure*; it is questionable whether tests on laboratory animals are of any value other than to weed out immediately lethal products. As one can not "prove a negative" it is impossible to prove that something is harmless.

Long-term ill effects have been reported from exposure to pesticides, heavy metals, volatile organic chemicals and "sick building syndrome" (in which the chemicals in the building are compounded by failure to clean the air conditioning ducts and contamination with mould spores occurs). From the domestic point of view, many new building and furnishing materials "off-gas" chemical vapours for at least nine months after installation (formaldehyde in particular). Anyone known to suffer with this problem should take very expert advice about materials before building or furnishing a house.

Many people with MCS develop chronic food allergy and candida problems as described above, and often benefit from help in tackling these problems, and reducing the "total load" even if nothing can be done to unwind the original chemical exposure. Avoidance of perfumes, alcohol and all chemicals as far as possible, is necessary, and is very difficult.

The diagnosis is made through taking a careful history and listening to the patient. There are no useful tests, yet, and physical examination does not help. Symptoms are often precipitated by very minor chemical exposures.

Symptoms of Multiple Chemical Sensitivity

- Energy loss
- Chronic fatigue
- Frequent 'flu like illnesses
- Depression/anxiety
- Increased sensitivity to light, sound, smell and pain
- Difficulty sleeping
- General irritability

Treatment

All the measures mentioned above for candida and mould will assist by reducing the "total load," avoidance of chemicals and unsuitable building and furnishing materials will help, also avoidance of all other unnecessary household chemicals and cosmetics, and only using a minimum of *unscented* products.

Other measures which can be helpful include chelation therapy, which has a mixed reputation, and two forms of immunotherapy: Enzyme Potentiated Desensitisation (EPD) and Provocative Neutralisation, (see chapter 5 for details). In some cases psychotherapy can help especially where there has been childhood or wartime trauma, but one must be clear that the patient's symptoms are *real*, and offer support and resolution for past trauma and current conflicts in conjunction with physical treatment, and not denial of the reality of the illness.

Chronic Fatigue Syndrome also known as Myalgic Encephalomyopathy (ME)

This is a collection of symptoms which follows a clearly defined virus infection, the most striking is profound muscular weakness, after even mild exertion. It seems to be much commoner in teenagers than it used to be. It is important to make the diagnosis (and distinguish it from drug addiction, eating disorders and depression) the treatment is as described above for reducing total load and intestinal candida, together with specialised advice and graded exercise to overcome the muscular problem. Geopathic stress, mobile phone masts and electrical phenomena in houses should also be considered. (Chapter 7)

Mumps Measles and Rubella (MMR) Vaccine Controversy

There is some "anecdotal" evidence from parents suggesting a connection between MMR and Attention Deficit Hyperactivity Disorder (ADHD) in children who were healthy before the vaccine was given and developed symptoms afterwards. The measures described above for environmental illness will all help by reducing the total load, some children will be greatly helped by mould precautions, and others by reducing the chemicals in their environment.

Waste Disposal ... An Allegory for our Times

Nothing changes. In olden times we threw sewage out of upstairs windows onto the roads and pavements below, and wondered why there was so much illness around. Later we understood, built sewers and invented hygiene.

Now we dump heavy metal waste, organophosphates and other detritus from our industrialised "civilisation" into the rivers and sea and onto the land whence it trickles into aquifers and water tables, and wonder why there is so much illness about. Will we never learn?

Chapter 9

Virus Infections and Shortening the Duration of a Cold

Viruses already play an increasing part in causing ill health, and with the current use of viruses as carriers for genes in the genetic manipulation of food and medicines, this could become a nightmare scenario, as we have no really effective antiviral drugs as yet. More recently the SARS virus illness has alarmed us and we are now facing the possible fall out from a 'flu virus in poultry which is apparently transmissible to man, especially those in close contact with infected chickens in the far east. World-wide air travel makes the possibility of a serious global epidemic very likely in the years to come.

Virus infections often precede environmental illness, especially Post Viral Syndrome but writing about the details will not help anyone to recover. Some of the general measures described in chapter 8 will help, as will the "Shortening a Cold" regime detailed here. I have noticed that colds are getting worse and lasting longer (mine and other peoples) and can only assume that the virus is changing and/or our "host resistance" is getting less efficient, perhaps through poor nutrition with industrialised and junk food.

Samways's Regime for Shortening the Duration of the Common Cold

The drug firms (producers of so many copycat and look alike drugs) have not, so far, produced anything to *cure* a common cold. They are already making a fortune selling palliatives that help minimally with the symptoms. The best I can offer is a regime of over-the-counter health products which have antiviral effects, and reduce the duration of a cold from two weeks to one week. (Rocket science.) Having said that, one needs to be very dedicated and stay at home, to carry out the regime. At this point we must distinguish a cold from 'flu which though very unpleasant, can be more easily treated.

A cold starts as a sore throat and is best treated at this point, which may prevent its further development. It goes on to runny/bunged up nose, cough and a feeling of near death, related to whatever is going on in the head. Loss of the voice is part of the deal, but one can usually walk about. It used to last 2 weeks, but nowadays may last much more and be called 'flu as that sounds better should time off work be needed, and it will, except for Trappist Monks; as any sustained effort at speech will result in a coughing fit which can not be hidden from clients etc.

For the purposes of this chapter, influenza ('flu) is different. The symptoms include cold and hot shakes, a terrible malaise and feeling of impending doom, joint and muscle pain and an urgent wish for death. The sufferer is in bed, not part of the world, and "if you stand up you fall down". The general anti-viral measures will do for both but 'flu can be treated by Neutralisation using dilutions of the 'flu vaccine (p49) this does not (usually) work for a cold as we have no extract of the cold virus.

A clinic specialising in Provocative Neutralisation will supply the 'flu vaccine and explain the process, which can "raise the dead" and get rid of 'flu symptoms in about an hour by stopping the body's allergic reaction to the virus. If planning this approach it is best to visit the clinic to be tested when well, and keep the vaccine in the fridge as clinics don't welcome the acutely infectious in their testing rooms.

Anti-viral Preparations to Shorten a Cold

Monolaurin (Chapter 18) 2 capsules four times daily. This works fastest if the powder is removed from the capsules, and swallowed from a spoon with water, otherwise the capsules may pass through the intestine expensively unchanged. Monolaurin is a prepararion of Lauric acid from coconuts and is a good anti-viral, it works by preventing the virus from replicating (breeding). For sore throat, the dose can be dissolved in the juice of an organic lemon, gargled and swallowed.

Oregano Oil capsules, 1 - 2 twice daily with food, swallow whole.

Zinc, other minerals and vitamins to taste, some people find **vitamin C** helps.

Colloidal Silver is an anti viral and is said to prevent colds, if only one knew in advance when one was going to get one. The dose on the bottle (usually 5ml three times daily) can safely be doubled. It can be used in a nebuliser for those who get chest infections, and as a nasal spray to aim for the sinuses. The downside is the cost. There are no side effects with any of these products.

Anas Barb Co 200 (Ainsworths, a homeopathic anti-viral remedy) taken under the tongue twice daily, away from food. One tablet taken weekly may help prevent virus infections.

Inhale steam several times a day using an electric steam inhaler, (Vick make a good one (p129)) which is designed to heat the steam to a temperature that will kill the virus. (A bowl of hot water will not work and its dangers may well contravene EU safety regulations.)

Keep taking the above regime for some days after symptoms have improved, otherwise it will all come back. Presumably it takes a while for the virus to be eliminated.

Comforters that do not Cure Anything:
Night Nurse Capsules 2 at bedtime (avoid the liquid, it contains alcohol) will stop all the nose and cough misery at night. Neither this nor Day Nurse capsules are curative but the latter can be used during the day to relieve symptoms; recently the capsules have been reformulated and they do not now contain phenylpropanolamine which causes raised blood pressure in some people and is best avoided. Day Nurse liquid should also be avoided as it contains alcohol.

Stay indoors as far as possible, and temporarily quit the exercise programme.

Food
Plenty of freshly juiced organic carrots, and other vegetables. Home made organic chicken soup, and anything else reasonably healthy that you fancy. Plenty of fluids.

Caveat: This regime is used by me and I find it helps, it has not undergone any clinical trials, so far as I am aware.

Chapter 10

Adult Children of Alcoholics and other Emotionally Challenged Families

Most doctors seem unaware of the long-term effects of chronic childhood trauma on the personalities and subsequent health of adults. Because of this (and because I specialise in treating these individuals) it is one of the chronic conditions included in this book. It is often the prelude to allergic conditions or Multiple Chemical Sensitivity (MCS) probably because the immune system was weakened by the daily fear and anxiety involved in surviving a traumatic childhood.

For brevity I include all those who had an emotionally, physically or sexually abusive childhood in this chapter. Most of the original work was done by Adult Children of Alcoholics (ACOAs), however other family addictions or secrets produce the same result, including gambling, philandering, workaholism, emotional absence, or over demanding parents, and so forth.

Since we only have one childhood, some people find it difficult to realise that their childhood was abusive as there is nothing with which to compare it. Normal parenting does not include frequent beatings, threats with guns, constant rowing and blaming, shouting and trashing the house (whether drunk or not). It does not include sexual abuse, boundary invasion, family secrets that are glaringly obvious and telling people that their feelings are wrong.

Case History

Janine, whose story was referred to under MCS (chapter 8), was brought up by a violent alcoholic father who regularly beat her younger brother when he (the father) came home drunk from the pub. He would start a scene and Janine was forced to watch all this without any power to intervene, and she learned to stuff her feelings especially anger and fear, inside from an early age. Apart from the violence, there was the family secret ("would daddy be ok?") so she could not safely bring her friends home. She did a lot of housekeeping and organising at a young age as her mother was a drudge and worked long hours to keep the family alcoholism going and never dared defend the children. The home atmosphere was rife with unspoken blame and misery. Later Janine said "it was the sheer daily-ness of the torture that was so terrible. It was like a war zone in which no-one knew who the enemy was."

Janine became a hard worker and did well at school in spite of the difficulties. She developed high standards and perfectionism, blamed herself for any shortcomings, felt almost permanently guilty and never good enough. She had a poor concept of interpersonal boundaries, took on other people's guilt and shame, and was unable to defend herself or voice her own needs. She later became something of a workaholic addictive salesperson, feeling, always, only as good as her last sale.

When she realised that her brother was big enough to defend himself physically, she left home and paid her way through business school by working as a waitress. After her diagnosis of MCS (chapter 8) she found a good therapist who helped her work through her childhood issues and encouraged her to attend meetings of a self-help group for people with similar problems. Eventually her physical and mental health improved and she learned to look after herself, say "no" ("No is a complete sentence... what is it that you don't understand about No?"). She divorced her alcoholic abusive husband and brought up her children in safety, although aware that they, in turn may later need help or even therapy, for past childhood abuse.

Janine's childhood was grossly abnormal, but there are much subtler degrees of emotional abuse which often go unrecognized, and unhelped.

The unwritten rule in an alcoholic family is "don't talk, don't trust, don't feel." This creed can last a life-time.

It is known that ACOAs tend to do any of the following more frequently than the rest of the population:

- Become alcoholic
- Marry alcoholics
- Develop other mental illness
- Develop serious physical illness

Family Dynamics of an Alcoholic Family

Roles

The Parents

Assuming only one parent is alcoholic (or a drug addict) the other parent will be the "chief enabler" who tries to hold the family unit together, goes to work to pay for alcohol (which is justified as earning to buy food, etc. but you can not ring-fence money) lies to cover up the drinking reality, hides drink, clears up the mess and on and on.

Addictive families revolve round the addict and the covering up involved, healthy families are flexible and do not revolve around one person. They are designed for the benefit of bringing up healthy children, not covering up unacceptable parental behavior. If both parents are alcoholic (or either is addicted to drugs) the chaos is even worse, and the downhill course quicker.

Children's Roles

These overlap and some people manage to play more than one role at different times, but the roles are illustrative.

The first child is the "hero" (Janine above), never feeling good enough inside, and highly efficient on the outside. Heroes try to redress the balance in a highly dysfunctional family. ("Keeping up appearances" and "someone's got to seem efficient round here".) Heroes tend to develop stress problems later on. They often join the healing or helping professions at which work they are very gifted after so much early training.

The second child is the "drop out", often a drug addict or alcoholic who perceives the impossibly high standards created by the first child and rebels rather than compete. Rebels often wind up in an addiction treatment unit (chapter 11) as chronic alcoholic/addicts or in trouble with the law.

The third child is the "lost child" who manages to disappear and not be noticed, who will read in a corner, be out of the house, or merge with the background.

The fourth child is the "clown" who tries to defuse the family malaise

71

with joking and clowning around, these children often become entertainers later on.

Under every hero there is a lost child, and that discovery is very painful. Most modern families do not have four children, so the roles may differ or combine somewhat.

Treatment

In an ideal world the whole family (including the dog) needs treatment, but that is rarely possible, so I treat those who are prepared to come, individually at first, and later several family members together.

Treatment for ACOAs and other Codependent Family Members

Consists of individual counselling and support, attendance at an appropriate self-help group and, if possible, attendance at residential or weekend workshops or specifically focused retreats.

Choosing a Therapist

Assuming reasonable qualifications, the most important thing about a therapist is *whether (or not) he/she has worked consistently and successfully on his/her own family of origin issues.* If they have not, then they will visit unresolved issues of their own onto the patient, and re-create yet another co-dependent family for the patient to fail to find their way out of. One should ask the therapist about their *own recovery* and whether they have a support group which they attend regularly. (See below.) The analogy I use is to ask myself the question do I think he/she (the therapist) "has climbed the Matterhorn?" A novice alpinist planning an ascent on the Matterhorn would be wise to choose a mountain guide who has done it before and knows the way, similarly it is best if the therapist has worked on their own emotional baggage.

No one is born emotionally "perfect," we all need an emotional "boot-camp" of some sort, one should find a therapist who attended a good one and worked hard and is still working on their emotional and spiritual growth and life-skills. Word of mouth recommendation through other sufferers may be best. There should be something optimistic and encouraging about a therapist's demeanour, and they should have a sense of humour and warmth.

Suitable Self-help Groups

People who got sick in a group (family) setting do best if part of their recovery activities are also in a group setting, where they can safely share their troubles and get the support of the group ("family of choice") for the behavioral changes they will have to make with their family of origin.

There are two kinds of group: those run by a therapist and usually requiring payment (avoid these; the therapist may be set up as Mummy or Daddy, if not Guru too...) and "Twelve Step Groups," so called because they are modeled on Alcoholics Anonymous, and use the same basic 12 Steps to recovery. These are "unled" groups, with no therapist, just the experience of other sufferers who have been in recovery longer and are further ahead on the road. The groups are usually held in church rooms and pass round a pot for small donations to cover the group's running costs. I can not overestimate the value of this latter approach. See also chapter 11 under AA. Any therapist who does not routinely refer patients to these groups should be avoided.

Twelve Step Self-Help Groups suitable for ACOAs and codependent family members include Codependents Anonymous (CODA) and Adult Children of Alcoholics (ACA or ACOA groups) the latter are an offshoot of Al Anon, which is for friends and families of alcoholics, but not specifically for *adult children* of alcoholics. If CODA and ACA/ACOA are not available in your area, then Al Anon will help educationally. Al Ateen is part of Al Anon for teenage children from alcoholic families. (See appendix 2 phone numbers.) These groups work on an anonymous basis, first names are used, and they meet weekly. The format of the meetings varies but often one person is designated to tell their story or lead a discussion on some aspect of recovery.

Workshops and Residential Treatment

All the caveats about choosing a therapist apply to choosing a workshop, especially as to the recovery status of those involved as therapists. My experience is that two centres in the USA run excellent residential workshops for ACOAs (there may be others.) They are Sierra Tucson in Arizona and Caron Foundation in Pennsylvania, mainly because of their insistence that all therapists and staff should have been through treatment for their own issues (p127).

Individual Therapy

My approach is gentle and initially slightly medical, endeavouring to establish trust by taking elementary details followed by a medical history and a description of the patient's presenting problem and worst difficulties. Over time we will visit the patient's childhood and discuss what happened in the light of the dysfunction of the parents, trying to get the blame off the patient who has been living with the feeling that "it was all their fault" for years. If sexual abuse occurred we will talk about this too, if possible. Perhaps the therapist's main function is to be a "safe person" and a good listener (rather than a "fixer"). Such people are rare in these families.

The construction of a family tree is useful, as it allows us to identify the addicts, alcoholics and just plain unpleasant people as well as certain talents in the family line. As this is also the starting point for enquiries about previous generations, it is helpful talk to the oldest person first and encourage them to reminisce about their childhood. The purpose is to find out what the unknown family members were like as people, and what special skills they had, some families denigrate their ancestors and the skills and talents get lost in the shuffle. The patient will have inherited some of these special gifts, and as a big part of therapy is to reclaim ones assets, their identification is a starting point.

Individual therapy should not last for ever, and is designed to deal with the worst of the problems, and to establish the patient in their self-help group so that this eventually becomes their on-going therapy. It is important to be aware that many ACOAs will develop food or environmental allergies and a candida problem *in recovery* (especially recovered alcoholics who also stop smoking,) and educate them as to the dietary approach to this.

Dream Workshops (chapter 19) can be helpful for those who continue to have recurrent nightmares. Doing a re-enactment of the scenario in a sympathetic and anonymous group sometimes stops the nightmares, or greatly reduces their frequency and horror quality.

Eating Disorders

Overeating, Anorexia Nervosa and Bulimia

These conditions often occur in co-dependent families particularly where the father is alcoholic, and there are high standards and a control-freak tendency.

The anorexics don't eat and are very thin, the bulimics binge and vomit (semi-secretly) and may be any size, but are often of normal weight.

The overeaters do just that and are often "career dieters" who know the calorific value of everything. Their eating which is about lack of self worth, involves sweet things and looks very like any other addiction. Recent research shows that some foods (chocolate, sugar) increase the "feel-good chemicals"(endorphins) produced by the brain. People with eating disorders of all kinds will benefit from attending Overeaters Anonymous, which is run along the same lines as AA.

Cynic's Corner

A wartime Admiralty safety instruction stated:

> *These mines must be stored with the bottom at the top: to avoid confusion, the top of the container has been marked "bottom".*

Living in an alcoholic family is a bit like that.

Chapter 11

Alcoholism and Addiction

My earlier comment about codependency being very poorly treated by conventional medicine, also applies to alcoholism and drug addiction. Unfortunately many doctors find the "pill fairy" irresistible. By the time alcoholics reach me they have usually been prescribed a tranquiliser by their GP. (Alcoholism is not a valium deficiency, giving a tranquiliser may make the alcoholic *smell* better, but it does nothing for their behaviour.)

The less fortunate will have seen a psychiatrist who may have changed the brand of tranquiliser and/or added an antidepressant, thus creating a pill problem too. Psychiatrists prefer to diagnose some other illness of the mind, which they can medicate; often manic-depression (bipolar illness); and patients and families buy into this. ("First class families don't get second class illnesses".) All this delays and worsens the real issue. Some specialists even now, pursue social drinking games, including asking drunken patients to keep drinking diaries, (which is a bit like learning navigation from the deck of a sinking ship, and bears no relation to reality.) We should be quite clear on one thing: alcoholics can not be made into social drinkers over any extended period of time. There is no such thing as an ex-virgin or an ex-alcoholic, but a *sober alcoholic can reconstruct their life.*

Case Histories

Peter was Janine's brother aged 29, (see pp69-70) he had been beaten and denigrated as a child by his alcoholic father, and believed life was hopeless. To escape his father he joined teenage gangs and used drugs including heroin, his behaviour at home became impossible, even by these family standards. He held menial jobs for short periods to pay for drugs and alcohol, was arrested and served prison sentences, and by the age of 24 he was in despair.

He was treated with out-patient therapy (individual counselling) as he was able to stop using drugs and alcohol at the hostel where he lodged which was a "dry house". He was supported while he became integrated into Alcoholics Anonymous, and has now been clean and sober for five years, and holds a job as a photographer. He has become an entirely different person and is getting married soon. He attended meetings of Narcotics Anonymous (NA) a self-help group for drug addicts for some years, too.

Joan was 65 when first seen, full of shame, she had an inherited title and high social standards. She lived alone as recluse with the vodka bottle as her only friend (thinking vodka doesn't smell, but it does) and had been caught shoplifting alcohol in her local supermarket, the publicity from which mortified her. She too was seen for individual therapy and support during which she became integrated into AA. Her daughter came for some family therapy and education about Alcoholism and attended Al Anon, a self-help group for the friends and family of those with alcohol problems.

Joan made a good recovery and is sober three years later, having re-established many of her old social contacts. She illustrates the point that women alcoholics are often much more secretive than men and tend to drink alone at home rather than in the pub, a trend that is changing now that so many young women are binge drinking in public places.

James was a 50 year-old solicitor who was in trouble at work as his partners had become aware of his drink problem, and he had a drink-driving charge pending. James was unwilling to come and did not initially realize the seriousness of the problem. However his wife came for help, and went, as suggested, to Al Anon for some months, whereupon James came for out- patient treatment. He too did very well in AA after a shaky start and a return to what he hoped would be social drinking, and which eventually proved to be disastrous. AA had indeed "spoiled his drinking."

Drug Addiction

Almost any drug may be abused by someone, so this table of drugs of addiction only gives an outline and a few examples of each group. The most abused drugs are those that produce artificial feelings of well being, or are stimulants (uppers) or sedatives (downers) or have hallucinogenic properties. There is also a miscellaneous group of substances which are inhaled, including volatile solvents (glue etc.) and anaesthetic gasses, abuse of the latter is usually confined to those with access through their work.

Table of Drugs of Addiction:

Narcotics (pain relievers)
- Heroin
- Morphine and other opiates
- Pethidine
- Diconal
- Methadone

Milder pain relievers commonly abused include
- Distalgesic
- DF 118
- Codeine mixtures in pills

Sleeping pills and Tranquilisers
- Barbiturates
- Valium and similar pills
- Temazepam and many others mainly ending in –azepam.
- Heminevrin

Stimulants (Uppers)
- Amphetamines
- Cocaine
- Appetite suppressants

Inhaled Volatile Substances
- Glue and solvents
- Anaesthetic gases

Halucinogens
- Canabis
- LSD
- PCB and a variety of other "street drugs"

Available over the counter
- Cough mixtures, especially codeine linctus
- Dr Collis Brown Mixture (chlorodyne.)

Drugs can be obtained from dealers or doctors. Methadone is

frequently supplied by psychiatrists running "harm reduction programs" together with needle exchanges in an attempt to prevent people sharing needles. Methadone is a heroin substitute and lacks the "high" the heroin addict is seeking, it can however be traded for money which can then, in turn, be used to buy heroin.

As methadone is long acting drug, it has long acting side effects and withdrawal symptoms, so my psychiatric colleagues are creating an addiction to a drug which is even more difficult to stop than heroin. Some of these doctors are a perfect example of the "Pusher Priest" and the more lavish prescribers are fortunately, now being brought to book. One has to question the motives of doctors who run *private* services that prescribe narcotics or sedatives to addicts on any basis that is longer than a supervised one week detox. programme. Narcotics addicts who truly wish to come off drugs can detoxify themselves using decreasing doses of codeine linctus purchased at the chemist, and many are aware of this, it takes only five days.

Drug addicts usually present for treatment at a younger age than alcoholics, their lifestyle having been even more disrupted, and inpatient detoxification may be needed to get them off drugs (especially if tranquilisers were used).

However since drug addicts abuse alcohol and alcoholics are nearly always involved in drugs (often from their GP) it is better to view addiction globally, and not get bogged down in details of amounts drunk or doses of drugs used (other than superficially on the first visit) but to be concerned about *behaviour*. It is the *combination of alcohol (or drugs) and trouble that makes the diagnosis*. Trouble tends to occur in any of the following areas of the person's life: finance, work, health, conflict with the law, domestic and family life, and deteriorating ethical values.

Indications for In-Patient Detoxification:

Alcoholics:
- Past history of DTs (Delirium Tremens) or fits when drying out.
- Unsuitable home circumstances.
- History of tranquiliser use.
- Co-existence of other health problems.
- Patient wishes to be an in-patient.

Drug Addicts:
- As above, plus lack of real motivation to stop.

Choice of Inpatient Rehabilitation Facility

There are basically two kinds:

Those run by psychiatrists and other therapists with a mental health background (avoid) and those run by recovered alcoholics who insist that their patients attend AA. (Recommended, provided well run.) Either can be NHS or fee-paying, most of the latter kind are privately run but take state-funded patients. Many private clinics have a few free places, but there is always a waiting list for these.

Any unit offering social drinking or "harm reduction" programmes is to be avoided. These just band-aid the real problem and do not offer rehabilitation to a changed and much improved life-style, which can only be achieved using a programme offering abstinence from alcohol and all mood altering drugs.

There are also some units with a strong Christian ethos and, while experience shows that sadly, God alone does not cure alcoholism, some of these centres can be a shelter for a person who needs to get away from home, or off the streets, and is able to combine the dry-house accommodation and religion with local AA meetings.

Most in-patient facilities keep people for only 30 days, but there are a number of half-way houses (dry houses with therapy) which form a stepping stone to normal life "outside".

Choice of Individual Therapist

The comments above on choosing a treatment unit also apply to therapists, the best choice would be a satisfactorily recovered alcoholic, with training and qualifications in counselling, who refers their patients to AA, rather than a psychiatrically trained individual who doesn't.

A family member (often the spouse) usually presents first, I prefer this, having found that a few detailed consultations with the sober family member seem to result in the alcoholic coming into some sort of treatment or AA, within about nine months or less. Part of the treatment for the family member is attendance at Al Anon meetings, and an explanation of how to stop "enabling" the alcoholic's drinking.

For example, pouring gin down the sink does not help, the alcoholic will have other bottles hidden, and it just adds to the cost. Covering up by telling his/her boss that he/she will not be in to work as they have 'flu or a funeral to go to ... again, only delays recovery, and fools nobody. It is best to do nothing and let the alcoholic sort it out when they wake up or sober up. Some times things have to get worse before they get better (Samways's Law: if something gets bad enough it eventually becomes "good".)

The alcoholic may come for treatment, in which case the initial motivation is usually to avoid the consequences of some alcohol-related disaster or other. The first consultation needs to be in the form of a history of what is going on at the time, together with a medical history and an assessment as to whether in-patient detoxification (dry-out) is medically indicated. Liver function and other blood tests and physical examination should be performed. Abnormal liver function tests are useful leverage that there is a medical (rather than "moral") problem with alcohol. However these tests are often normal except in late stage alcoholism or briefly, after a major binge.

Drinking histories should be about events and consequences, rather than an exercise in counting drinks and bottles which is invariably inaccurate. Some therapists distinguish between binge drinkers ("periodics") and daily drip-feed drinkers, but in truth, the binges get closer together and more disastrous with time, and abstinence is the only answer. Binge drinkers may wonder why they need AA when they are not drinking, and at an early stage may be harder to treat. The modern trend of urban weekend, pub and club binge drinking with drugs in young people, may well lead to an increase in alcoholism later. One should distinguish between temporary drunkenness and alcoholism which is long term. However one may lead to the other.

Alcoholics Anonymous (AA) was started in America by two alcoholics in the nineteen thirties, it is a self-help group with meetings in most towns and districts in the English speaking world. There are no chiefs, everyone is in recovery, some longer than others. Officers rotate and first names are used. Meetings vary and it is important for the newcomer to find meetings they like, but the therapist should be aware that, initially they may not like any as they do not wish to go at all. I usually point out (at the stage of "but I don't like AA …") that he/she doesn't have to like it, diabetics may not like their diet or insulin … He/she is just asked to go.

A diabetic needs to attend to his insulin, blood tests and diet, in order to stay well, if he does this he can lead a relatively normal life. Likewise the alcoholic needs to attend to his sobriety by going to meetings, and following the AA recovery programme of 12 Steps. He will need to get a sponsor (someone with some years of sobriety, who is willing to act as teacher and guide, and of the same sex,) and later will learn how to pass on the message to other drinking alcoholics. If he does this and gains the social skills of refusing drinks firmly and without normally causing offence, he can lead a normal life.

Alcoholics who do not go to AA usually do not get sober (dry of alcohol and off all mood-altering drugs). If they do achieve abstinence they do not usually change their mindset and so become "dry drunks" who are tetchy and difficult to have around and often develop stress related physical illnesses or other addictions (gambling, food, sex) later on. Recovery is a real but slow process that does not happen in isolation, at home in front of the TV.

It is useful for the doctor or therapist to have a list of former patients in good recovery who are willing to help newcomers, and with the consent of the newcomer, phone the old-timer and ask them to make contract, and take the new person to a meeting. The choice of former patient is important, they should be of the same sex and if possible, and of similar social background, as this will provide commonality of purpose and reduce stigma. For example, a solicitor helping another lawyer or accountant gives the unspoken message that professional people, and not just vagrant meths. drinkers, do recover from alcoholism. Helping newcomers is referred to as "Twelfth Stepping" (from the wording of the last of AA's Twelve Steps) and helps both parties involved.

Sponsorship

Initially everyone is advised to find a sponsor, and the above comments about social background and sex also apply, with the exception that a gay or lesbian person might choose a sponsor of the *opposite sex*, to minimise distractions.

A sponsor, often initially referred to as a "caretaker-sponsor" to allow for change if it doesn't work; is someone with at least two years sobriety who is prepared to help the newcomer with the recovery program in detail. Both parties gain immensely from the exercise, and a lot of coffee is consumed. The newcomer should choose a sponsor who has something attractive about their recovery, and may need to take advice from the older members of their group. People do "out-grow" sponsors and may need to make a change later on.

The AA Recovery Programme

This is based on the 12 Steps of AA (page84) and there are books available to explain the details. Reference to God or a Higher Power does *not* imply any specific religion, the alcoholic can choose any God of their understanding or none, atheists often do very well provided they come to believe that *they* are not God.

The steps start with an admission of powerlessness over alcohol and the unmanageability of life. Then there is a statement that a belief in a Higher Power (anything from God to a teapot, not necessarily God as in religion) can restore sanity; and a decision to hand many of the more imponderables of life over to that Higher Power, and drop the control-freak tendency.

Next come two steps involving a personal inventory of the deficiencies and excesses of the drinking saga, and a sharing of this with "God" and another person, which helps with guilt and shame. This is followed by the making of lists of character defects and assets, and of people harmed during the drinking years, together with a resolve to make amends wherever possible. Amends include an effort *not* to repeat the offending behaviour, and go much further than an apology alone.

The final three steps are a continuation of the inventory on a daily basis to sort things out as they occur, a continuing effort to grow in spiritual values including prayer and meditation, a resolve to help others with the same problems, and to practice the principles embodied in the AA Twelve Steps in general life.

The newcomer to AA will learn that they are not alone, they have an illness rather than moral turpitude, that will-power alone doesn't work, and that social or controlled drinking is not an option. (If it was, they wouldn't need to be at AA or seeking professional help.)

Without wanting to complicate the issue that abstinence and attendance at AA are the primary goals in early recovery, those who have some months of sobriety may develop food allergy and candida problems (see chapters 3,4 and 5) and would do well to look at the dietary approach suggested, and ensure the mineral and vitamin deficiencies concomitant with alcoholism or drug addiction are corrected by supplementation and good quality food.

"Alcohol gave me wings to fly
Then it took away the sky."

(Alcoholics Anonymous, Big Book)

The 12 Steps of Alcoholics Anonymous

1   We admitted we were powerless over alcohol—that our lives had become unmanageable.

2   Came to believe that a Power greater than ourselves could restore us to sanity.

3   Made a decision to turn our will and our lives over to the care of God as we understood Him.

4   Made a searching and fearless moral inventory of ourselves.

5   Admitted to God, to ourselves, and to another human being the exact nature of our wrongs.

6   Were entirely ready to have God remove all these defects of character.

7   Humbly asked Him to remove our shortcomings.

8   Made a list of all persons we had harmed, and became willing to make amends to them all.

9   Made direct amends to such people wherever possible, except when to do so would injure them or others.

10 Continued to take personal inventory and when we were wrong promptly admitted it.

11 Sought through prayer and meditation to improve our conscious contact with God as we understood Him, praying only for knowledge of His will for us and the power to carry that out.

12 Having had a spiritual awakening as the result of these steps, we tried to carry this message to alcoholics, and to practice these principles in all our affairs.

AA 12 Steps and 12 Traditions

Reprinted with the permission of The General Service Board of Alcoholics Anonymous (Great Britain) Limited

Chapter 12

Allergy and Addiction – the Crossover

As a doctor working with both addicts and allergics over many years, I have noticed certain commonalities and overlap between the two illnesses, and have developed some theories about mechanisms and causation, as well as treatment ideas.

I will give my own definitions of addiction and allergy, there are many versions of this.

Addiction

The chronic repetitive ingestion of a substance, or the persistent repetition of an activity that originally caused a "high" or improvement in feelings. With this goes the belief that the addictant (substance or action) will do so again and again. In English, I mean that recurrent use of substances such as alcohol or drugs or the repeated unhealthy use of some activities (including gambling, sex, shopping, computers and work) can lead first, to a high, later a staving off of withdrawal symptoms and finally, to ongoing harm and despair. Food comes into this list, it is an ingested substance, but the behavioural nature of this addiction makes it look more like an activity addiction.

With addiction "tolerance" develops over time, which means that the addict requires an increasing dose of the substance or frequency of the activity concerned, in order to maintain a reasonable state of mind. By this stage they will not reliably get a "high" off their addictant, but will be using it in a futile endeavour to stay normal and stave off withdrawal symptoms.

Withdrawal symptoms occur when the addict does not get the next "fix" in time and the symptoms can be stopped temporarily by another dose of the addicting substance or activity.

Withdrawal Symptoms Include:

- Cold Shakes and 'flu like symptoms
- Profound weakness

- Panic, fear, anxiety and depression
- Feeling of impending doom and inability to cope
- Nausea, vomiting, diarrhoea and abdominal pain
- Runny nose and much else.

Allergy

This might be defined as an illness or set of unpleasant symptoms caused by the ingestion into the body of one or more substances (which may be eaten, breathed or absorbed through the skin). The reaction may be acute (nuts etc) or chronic as in food and inhalant allergies. Once sufferers become aware of the cause they will avoid it like the plague.

Perhaps the opposite of tolerance may occur in some people who seem to get more sensitive to their allergic substance with time and inadvertent exposure. Shell fish allergy and wasp stings may be examples of this, though the mechanism is different from that of chronic food allergy often related to intestinal yeast overgrowth.

The symptoms of allergy may be any or all from the above list of withdrawal symptoms from addiction, with the addition of:

- Bloating of the abdomen (stomach)
- Swelling of feet and ankles
- Obesity unresponsive to diet.

Perhaps withdrawal from addiction is really an allergic reaction in the way that some allergies can be "turned off" by a neutralising dose of the allergen (see chapter 5 allergy shots). Certainly I have heard a medical colleague publicly propound the theory that alcoholism is merely a food allergy to the rye or potatoes from which the alcohol was made. (Don't try it, recovered folk – treating alcoholism really does require abstinence.)

I doubt if anyone really understands the cellular mechanisms involved in allergy or addiction, the brain chemistry experts are the best bet for the future. I have considered why there are so many people who have suffered from both, and especially the almost universal occurrence of candida, mould and food allergy problems in addicts and alcoholics who are in recovery and no longer "using". Of course it is possible that these people had allergy symptoms when they were taking drugs or alcohol and didn't notice them, as "one doesn't notice a fleabite under a general anaesthetic." The allergy and candida symptoms tend to occur after several month of abstinence. (Being clean and dry.)

My conclusion is that there are basic underlying causes that weaken the immune system in childhood and persist in adult life. Most addicts come from family backgrounds that included emotional or other abuse in childhood and believed they were "not good enough" (see chapter 10). I suspect they suffered chronic fear as children; fear spread thin on a daily basis. We are designed for fight or flight, acute reactions to major fear from sudden events. This produces adrenaline, cortisone and other stress chemicals in the body to aid in the chosen form of escape. In many families fight or defiance is not possible, and all the anger, fear and associated feelings are stuffed down inside (food does a great job at this) and as the feelings are not dissipated, they rumble on internally along with the stress chemicals that were never used up. I suspect this weakens the immune system on a long-term basis.

People recovering from co-dependency issues also tend to develop these problems, and the childhood origin is obvious. Many patients who come to me for allergy problems are found to have a similar childhood history to those mentioned above, and some have the early stages of substance or other addiction. Finally the alcoholics in recovery will have had a major exposure to the yeast component involved in the fermentation of alcohol, which encourages candida and yeast overgrowth, and a diet that we probably deficient in proper nutrients.

Some years ago, while visiting a unit specialising in co-dependency and childhood issues, I happened to ask a very wise doctor about the allergy connection, and he replied, "candida is really a boundary issue". What he meant was that, in the same way that we seem powerless to stop some people from making impossible demands which we feel we must obey, people with gut candida overgrowth problems have got, symbolically, the same problem inside, as outside. There is an element of truth in this, as, when the childhood boundary issue of inability to say "no" (remember: "no" is a complete sentence) is gradually overcome, along with the guilt that goes with it, the candida problem seems to improve. Perhaps this is just due to stress reduction, but it certainly helps.

Unfortunately the fragmentation of medicine is such that the doctors who see and treat addiction (often psychiatrists) are not usually the doctors who see allergy (at best allergy specialists, sometimes other generalists or immunologists) who usually miss the childhood co-dependency component of allergy and its weakening effect on the immune system. It seems that each only treats "their half" with limited results. My approach takes in both the lingering childhood destructive messages and the allergy and environmental components of this complex illness.

There are very few allergy specialists in the UK and most of these run private services, as the NHS has not caught up with allergy as a major cause of expense and ill health. The same is true of addiction, only the government approach here is a hand-wringing exercise involving statistics, rather than any real effort to set up abstinence-based treatment centres which are badly needed. Addiction causes financial losses on a truly industrial scale, it is very often missed and treated as something else.

Chapter 13

Staying Healthy in Later Life and Avoiding the Pill Fairy

All the guidelines for healthy eating, candida and mould control mentioned earlier in this book and the Hay Diet, will help in a general way. Nutritional supplements especially minerals are important. (See chapter 18.) Eating Organic food will minimise the intake of toxic chemicals, the long-term effects of which, in untested combinations, are unknown and unlikely to be harmless. Organic food can not be genetically modified or irradiated.

Other problems: Have a thyroid function test done periodically. Joint pains and arthritis often improve dramatically after dealing with mould (Chapter 5.)

Get a Juicer and make vegetable juice from *organic* vegetables, drink immediately, it loses its vitamins and "life-force" if left to stand. Carrots are excellent (in theory one may turn orange if overdosing on carrot juice) and most other vegetables will be of benefit. Root vegetables are surprisingly good. Fruit is also good but beware of too much sugar (which encourages candida growth.) L'Equip make a robust juicer at a reasonable price (p129).

Hormone Replacement Therapy

I am ambivalent about HRT, but it has a place where health problems arise at, or soon after, the menopause. These may include intractable palpitations and flushes, also depression and anxiety problems. There are two kinds of HRT:

Hormones available from the Medical Profession (on the NHS). These may be made from processed mares' urine or synthetically. Hormones come as a pill, patch, implant or cream and have a variety of constituents and combinations. They usually aim to provide extra oestrogen, primarily. **Natural Hormone Replacement Therapy** so called because it is not made from mares' urine, but from a plant molecule which is identical, or very similar to, human hormones. It is available from American compounding pharmacies who make up a prescription individually for each patient, following analysis of a saliva sample which shows which hormones (including DHEA from the adrenals) are low and need boosting. Saliva tests can be repeated periodically to check on progress and point to any alterations needed in the hormone mix. This form of HRT comes as a cream to be rubbed into the skin, and is a much more logical approach to the problem in the long term.

The proponents of natural HRT suggest that long-term oestrogen treatment causes problems including raised blood pressure, and that progesterone (with or without DHEA as capsules) may be a better option, in later life and for the long term. This is claimed to be as effective in preserving bone density. The real snag is the cost. It can be obtained by post. (See chapter 19 and appendix 2.)

Bone Density

Avoiding osteoporosis (bone thinning) is one of the intended functions of HRT. Some families show a genetic tendency to osteoporosis and menopausal women from these might consider the use of some form of HRT. However my comments on good nutrition together with suitable daily regular exercise will assist in maintaining good bone structure. Adequate calcium is essential as part of a balanced mineral intake, but some experts think that calcium supplements alone lead to harder, more brittle bones which break more easily.

Regular Exercise

It is easier to keep fit then to get fit after a period of inactivity, therefore I recommend at least twenty minutes of sensible exercise daily, swimming, walking or cycling being the least likely to cause impact injuries or otherwise stress aging joints. Cycling can be on the road or by exercise bike, but since the latter is mind-numbingly boring, it can be combined with talking books or music borrowed from the Public Library. Swimming is best done by time rather than counting lengths, as one can then use the brain for other things (like writing this book) which makes it more interesting and purposeful. The most important thing about choice of exercise is that you should enjoy it.

I find it useful, occasionally, to remember that our ancestors were hunter-gatherers and would have spent all day either hunting or gathering, ie. walking with occasional bursts of sprinting either to kill prey or to escape from a predator. Presumably we were designed to thrive on this regime and in cultures where hunter gathering is still a way of life, they have no word in their vocabulary for "exercise," as no one in their right mind would exercise after eight hours of hunter-gathering.

In this connection I have often wondered if part of the appeal of shopping is related to some deeply ingrained need to search for items which we can store now to enhance our life for later on. (So the fantasy goes ...)

Athletic fitness is not the same as being healthy. There are plenty of healthy people who could not begin to run a marathon, and plenty of "fit" athletes who suffer from chronic ill-health and injury because of a combination of poor nutrition and over-exercise, which tend to lower their immune system and result in recurrent infections.

Blood Pressure

If blood pressure is taken and found to be raised, it should be measured several times over a period of days after the person has been sitting quietly. If it is still raised, a trial of a "self-take" blood pressure machine should be done at home, if possible. This eliminates the stress cum white coat syndrome which leads to false high readings. The patient should take their blood pressure in the morning and evening and record the results. If truly raised, a trial of minerals and vitamins may help, if all else fails a small dose of a beta-blocker such as atenolol can be tried, with continued monitoring at home and discussion of the results with the doctor.

All the usual causes of raised blood pressure should first be addressed, these include smoking, alcohol consumption, overweight and stressful lifestyle. But also (see below) beware! The so-called "normal range" is, for no obvious reason other than finance, being lowered. In any case, the normal range of blood pressure for someone over the age of sixty, especially fit women with no family history of heart problems, is a moot point.

Pros and Cons of Screening (Health Check-ups) in Later Life:

Having worked for the UK's major health screening company for 17 years I have seen both sides of this question and undoubtedly annual screening involving a good physical examination by an experienced doctor together with tests such as cervical smear, mammography and blood-work can lead to early diagnosis of cancer and other illnesses. Also advice on lifestyle and diet may be useful. The downside is more complicated, including such unanswered questions as whether the radiation from annual mammograms added to the body's total radiological load could, over time, be a contributory cause of cancer; whether "breast (cancer) awareness" and the regular self-examination of breasts may unconsciously or in some not yet understood way, actually encourage the development of breast cancer.

The current advice on lowering cholesterol is questionable in the light of such books as "The Cholesterol Myths" by Uffe Ravnskov. It is unlikely that dietary fat restriction actually lowers blood cholesterol very much, and even less likely that such lowering is actually beneficial. Now there is a move to lower the values of the normal range for blood pressure, which will "pathologise" a whole new group of otherwise normal people, into the profitable net of those unnecessarily prescribed BP lowering pills.

As medical students, we were taught about logical falsehoods and wrong conclusions, using the example: "my cat has four legs, my table has four legs … therefore my cat is a table". Something similar may have occurred with the old observation that *some families* suffer from raised cholesterol levels and the early onset of heart disease. This was not necessarily cause and effect and may be an inherited tendency affecting *these* families.

The current state of prostate cancer screening is unsatisfactory. Although we have tests, the results are often unclear, and can not yet distinguish which prostate cancers will be invasive and need treatment, and which will stay in the prostate and not need treatment. (The treatment is not a minor matter here.)

Finally good screening is expensive. There is some logic in having a screen every ten years starting at age 40 and stopping around the age of sixty. A regular thyroid function test and other blood tests from ones GP would be cheaper and less of an ordeal.

Keep the Brain Cells Active

Regular enjoyable mental exercise will keep the brain active, suggestions include doing cryptic crosswords, learning to play Bridge, other card games, reading and joining a literature or book group, participating in amateur dramatics (electricians, seamstresses and many other backstage skills are also needed, so inability to act is no bar), starting a discussion group and so on. Again it is important to choose something you enjoy and best if it is done with other people. Research shows that those who keep a pet and/or attend regular events with other people, seem to have a better chance of staying healthy in old age.

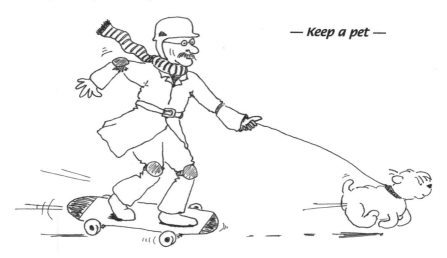

— Keep a pet —

Have a Purpose in Life

After retirement it is easy to lose ones purpose or direction. One way of avoiding this is to become involved in voluntary work in an area in which one is interested. This means participation either on the committee or as a regular worker. One can also support the charity financially rather than the scattergun approach of giving to all those who call at the door rattling tins. Seeing a small charity with worthy aims become a national force for good is very rewarding.

The Skin Horse

From The Velveteen Rabbit by Margery Williams

The Skin Horse had lived longer in the nursery than any of the others. He was so old that his brown coat was bald in patches and showed the seams underneath, and most of the hairs in his tail had been pulled out to string bead necklaces. He was wise, for he had seen a long succession of mechanical toys arrive to boast and swagger, and by-and-by break their mainsprings and pass away, and he knew that they were only toys, and would never turn into anything else. For nursery magic is very strange and wonderful, and only those playthings that are old and wise and experienced like the Skin Horse understand all about it.

"What is REAL?" asked the Rabbit one day, when they were lying side by side near the nursery fender, before Nana came to tidy the room. "Does it mean having things that buzz inside you and a stick-out handle?"

"Real isn't how you are made," said the Skin Horse. "It's a thing that happens to you. When a child loves you for a long, long time, not just to play with, but REALLY loves you, then you become Real."

"Does it hurt?" asked the Rabbit.

"Sometimes," said the Skin Horse, for he was always truthful. "When you are Real you don't mind being hurt."

"Does it happen all at once, like being wound up," he asked, "or bit by bit?"

"It doesn't happen all at once," said the Skin Horse. "You become. It takes a long time. That's why it doesn't happen often to people who break easily, or have sharp edges, or who have to be carefully kept. Generally, by the time you are Real, most of your hair has been loved off, and your eyes drop out and you get loose in your joints and very shabby. But these things don't matter at all, because once you are Real you can't be ugly, except to people who don't understand."

"I suppose you are real?" said the Rabbit. And then he wished he had not said it, for he thought the Skin Horse might be sensitive. But the Skin Horse only smiled.

"The Boy's Uncle made me Real," he said. "That was a great many years ago; but once you are Real you can't become unreal again. It lasts for always."

Chapter 14

Spiritual Growth and the Purpose of Life

Few people embark on "spiritual growth" voluntarily, usually it is forced upon them as part of recovery from serious illness or some other devastating and life-changing event. It involves major alterations in life-style and values, and is infinitely rewarding later on. Some people achieve this through their church, but the majority do not and find their own path through books, teachers and other methods. "Life is a journey, not a station you stop at."

The churches seem to have limitations in respect of their emphasis on money, power and control, to which end a feeling of guilt and shame is instilled with God or the priest as "Celestial Policeman." Most people who try to follow this path are already full of guilt, shame and a pervasive feeling of life-long inadequacy and of never having been "good enough" at which point they look elsewhere. Fortunately there are books and organisations which have embraced the best bits of many religions which can be very helpful in providing rules and guidance through that minefield we call daily life.

I have come to believe that life is a kind of celestial boot camp or training ground, and that there is a continuation of the soul or spirit after this. Many people take the view that we agreed to certain challenges in this life (before birth) and then tore up the rulebook or recipe, so that we have no idea what we came here to achieve. (One can find out bits of the latter by a dedicated quest.)

Four Stages of Spirituality:

Scott Peck in "Further Along the Road Less Travelled" describes four stages of spiritual development, I have summarised his four stages, which are a very good way of looking at people and families:

Stage 1: Chaos.
Unmanageable lives varying from criminality through addiction, cruelty, victim-hood to abuse and abused. "Most people lead lives of quiet

desperation." However chaos is rarely "quiet".

Stage 2: Spirituality within walls.

People who cope well with life where there are strongly enforced outside rules, including those who thrive in the military and in prison and who fail to cope outside but are recurrent, but model, prisoners. Also there are those who do well in strict religious circumstances, but are at sea without the rules and regulations enforced from outside. Stage two is where most people in the churches stay. It is an awful lot better than stage one, but fraught with anxiety, and works through fear of being found out or found deficient.

Stage 3: Rebellion.

If the stage two people go into therapy (for childhood or other issues) they will eventually enter a stage of anger and rebellion against the "walls" and what happened therein. This is healthy, although the person may not be a bundle of laughs while they are going through this stage and blaming everyone in sight. It is a process and takes time.

Stage 4: Mysticism.

(There are several stages of mysticism too.) The person has grown through the rebellion, confronted what happened and their part in it, made amends, forgiven those concerned and themselves, and learned to live differently, including setting sensible boundaries with others and dealing with anger appropriately.

The mystic will do many of the things required of those within walls, but on an entirely voluntary basis because they wish to, or feel better if they do. The will have a sort of unobtrusive internal discipline and are not trying to please some outside celestial policeman. Their lives will, to the outsider, look effortless, and will run much more smoothly and attractively than those of people in the first three stages. They will have learned to keep relatively quiet about some things.

Stage four looks a little like stage two, but is without any outside compulsion. People in stage two are often frightened to death by people in stage four. Stage three, rebellion, may look a bit like stage one, chaos. Rebellion is the process by which people grow through their past pain and blame and on to better things, chaos is usually going nowhere, unless there is a crisis which is used for advancing to stage two.

For example, an alcoholic in the depths of despair in stage one goes to an enlightened doctor, who refuses to play the tranquiliser game, and tells the alcoholic to go to AA. Initially he finds the rules (i.e. 12 Steps and group behaviour), enforced loosely from outside, and gets sober. Later he confronts his family and childhood issues with a therapist, goes through rebellion and eventual healing and on to stages of mysticism, and keeps on growing spiritually *because he wants to*. This whole process will take about ten years of daily sustained but pleasant effort which eventually becomes a comfortable way of life.

What they did Not Teach us at School

The following comments about childhood trauma should be looked at in the light of ones <u>own</u> childhood, and <u>not</u> in the light of ones efforts at parenting ones children. All parents do their best, no one can change what they have done as a parent, but we can change our outlook and eventually the mental health issues resulting from our own childhood trauma. No, it was not your fault, but if the results are a daily fact of life, the problem must be addressed or it will continue to cause pain. The buck stops here.

Many people seem to start life with a feeling of inadequacy, I call this original shame, to be distinguished from original sin, which implies that we did or failed to do something, whereas original shame just is.... The origins are in our upbringing, and the parental tendency to criticise. It is important to be clear that certain *behaviour* is bad or unwanted, but the person (child) is *not* bad or unwanted. It is also vital to be affirmative and say so when something is good or has been done well.

Self-esteem (self-worth) is a huge subject, and lack of it (fear spread thin) is at the root of most human misbehaviour and addictions. Self esteem in adult life can be improved by various forms of individual and group therapy including self-help groups, and by specific workshops designed to tackle the original causes, which may result from child abuse, including emotional, physical and sexual abuse.

Learning to Set Boundaries

It is important to know where "I leave off and you begin," in the physical sense and emotionally. We all know when our physical boundaries are being invaded, perhaps by someone who stands just that bit too close for comfort (and has, if we are unlucky, the sort of bad breath that would strip paint) so one backs off, and they step up in a sort of grisly pas de deux, until eventually one is backed up against the wall with nowhere to go.

Emotional boundaries are more subtle and sometimes the clue is a vague feeling of unease. Examples include those who dump their emotional baggage upon other people, make unreasonable (and non-negotiable) demands, use subtle forms of blackmail, criticism or victim-hood to gain their own ends and anyone who ever comes up to you and says "you are not looking well, is anything the matter?" If you are ill you know it, and if you are not ill, you don't want to hear about it; this is usually a put down, and *not* caring.

Avoid taking on other peoples emotional baggage, if someone is bad tempered in the office, it is most likely to be their problem and not something you did or said. Also avoid invading other people's boundaries, some people are natural boundary invaders, perhaps because they had an unavailable parent whose attention could only be gained by prodding them in the ribs (actually or metaphorically). Equally do not expect others to divine your needs, some things do need to be asked for, people whose parents were restrictive ("it's wrong to have needs") or invasive, usually have problems voicing their own needs, however basic. People who have boundary issues often marry abusive spouses, and then compound and repeat the problem.

Remember "No" is a complete sentence. "… and what is it that you don't understand about no?"

Other people's loud music (and its piped equivalent in public places) is an invasion of boundaries (as is other people's cigarette smoke) but these seem to be "generally acceptable" and it is difficult to protest. However the Campaign Against Piped Music (p127) which deals with piped music in public places, not nuisance neighbour's noise, is worth joining if badly affected. Some people "don't hear" piped music, so they say, and are not bothered by it.

In restaurants I always ask that the music be turned *off* ("down" or "quietly" are not expressions that are understood any more) while indicating that I will tip better for silence and am somewhat deaf (all done politely). If that fails, I explain and leave, as I shall not enjoy an evening of banging noise, however good the food, and conversation will be impossible. Since writing this, I have discovered why it is so hard to persuade staff to turn off piped music: *because it is being played for the benefit of the staff* (often younger) and not for the customers, who are often older and hate it, but lack the guts to say so.

Time and energy are, in a sense, boundary issues, since one may run out of either of them, but energy can usually be revived by having a break or inserting regular breaks into ones diary, and avoiding being too busy to enjoy things. Running on "flat batteries" is not a good idea for any length of time.

Anger

This is a very common problem, and as a society we do not deal with it very well. Anger is a feeling, it is not good or bad, it just is. What we do with it is vital. If we hit our neighbour over the head with a machete we will go to gaol, so what we do with our anger has consequences. If we stuff it or deny it, it will have consequences for health including substance addiction, high blood pressure and other stress related illnesses. Anger needs to be dealt with rationally, which is difficult when angry. It was originally designed to enable us to fight or flee when confronted by a wooly mammoth on the Serengeti. Life is rather different now.

Causes of anger can broadly be divided into two categories: ones needs not being met and invasion of boundaries. When feeling angry it is worth sitting down and thinking about the cause, and what one would like done to resolve the problem. If it started in the supermarket check-out queue, when the woman behind, with the mountain of fast food and cartel of free range children; ran her trolley over your feet; you have a choice, either say something, or to let it go, *you will probably never see her again.* It is the recurrent problems with the same people (usually family or work mates) that really need sorting out.

The hard bit is to work out a solution to the problem and then discuss it rationally with the other person, when you both have the time, energy and privacy to discuss it properly (not when a spouse has just walked in tired from a long days work, and not when someone has been using alcohol or drugs). The solution will probably be a compromise. If there is a really recurrent problem which has resulted in many broken promises to change, the person affected may have to think of radical solutions, and should seek advice, first from trusted friends.

If anger is out of all proportion to what triggered it, then it is related to childhood issues, and not really to the apparent trigger. I call this "original rage", it usually needs some form of therapy and, untreated, may lead to domestic or other violence.

99

Control Issues

Some people seem to have a need to control everything, including other people to a pathological degree. Others are compulsive supervisors (Margot in the TV programme "The Good Life"). It is unwise ever to sit down in their presence. Living with a control-freak is hell. In truth very little can be controlled, and never other people. One can, however take control of ones own life, to some extent anyway. It is a mistake to surrender control to authority figures or to family members, which comes back to setting boundaries, and learning, by experience, what is reasonable and acceptable behaviour.

Belief in a Higher Power

Many people develop some form of faith in a higher power either through their religion or by another route. I found the "celestial policeman" approach of the churches unsatisfactory and over many years of study have come to believe in a God of Nature, with a Universal Purpose. Anyone who has stood and looked at the stars at night or the sea or any other scene of Nature will have little difficulty in believing that whatever is going on, we are pretty small by comparison. There is a "Power greater than oneself" out there. Over time and with spiritual growth, ones faith in this power strengthens and some of the concepts change and deepen.

Prayer and Meditation

Whether, or not one believes in God or a higher power, the regular practice of prayer, meditation and reading spiritual books (a bit at a time, daily) will improve the quality of life. These practices encourage belief where none originally exists, and at the very least, if carried out morning and evening, will provide a quiet time to plan the new day or go over the events at the end of the old one, and decisions about things forgotten or needing attention can be made. This is meditation at its most basic, and it is a tool for effective living.

Prayer can be part of this; for oneself, other people, the sick and all those in need. It may be wiser to pray "for people" (perhaps to have the strength to cope) or for the "general good" rather than for a specific outcome to someones illness or problem. The real benefit comes from making this a regular discipline and part of ones daily life, which it will enhance. In the morning, set the alarm about 20 minutes early, initially this is a shock to the system, but it will soon become part of an indispensable routine. An evening session can be incorporated into ones bedtime activities.

Rules for Living

It is helpful to have a code of general behaviour, and many religions provide one, even if some of the surrounding baggage dilutes or confuses the issue. The 12 steps of AA (or CODA or Al Anon) p84 provide an excellent guide to living, including the making of amends for past mistakes, and the removal of the worst character defects.

Here are some guidelines for life from my experience:

1   Be a "generalist" rather than a specialist. Become reasonably competent in a wide range of activities and you will have much more fun than the narrow specialist. (Who, at a party, talks for long to the nuclear physicist or quantity surveyor with no social skills?)

2   Learn to drive a car well, it is the most dangerous thing most of us do regularly after the age of 50. Take an advanced driving course, including skid pan skills, concentrate and make allowances for other peoples errors, it may save your life.

3   Learn about food, nutrition, the environment and your body, become an expert on your own needs for health. Avoid conventional doctors and drugs as far as possible. Notice what aberrations the food industry is quietly foisting on us, such as which foods can be genetically modified or irradiated, and avoid them.

4   Make friends, acquire good social skills including the ability to set boundaries and say "no" when appropriate.

5   Have fun, very few people die regretting that they didn't spend more time washing dishes or rodding drains.

6   Invent your own rules.

Remember:

Life Should have Choices Beyond Mere Survival.
Life is a journey, not a station you stop at.

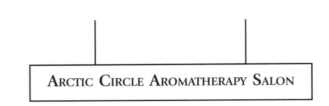

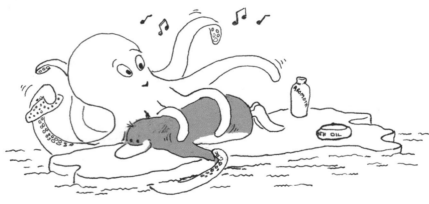

— *"Feel Good Factor"* —

Chapter 15

On Dying Well at Home

There are only two certainties in life, death and taxes. Most of us devote more time to avoiding both of these, than to considering the inevitability of death and how to "die well", preferably at home. The latter takes very specific organisation.

First one must develop some kind of philosophy of life which accepts death either as part of an ongoing process, and not total annihilation, or take some other view, otherwise it is difficult to consider it reasonably comfortably and make sensible plans. This philosophy should include a good quality diet and lifestyle in an endeavour to stay fit and keep out of the hands of the doctors, who regard death not as a natural process, but as a failure of their mission and therefore something to be fought off at all costs.

Doctors are useful for pain and symptom relief, but there the matter usually ends. It is sadly true that many doctors in their *professional capacity, do not experience the process of death in its entirety* with the emotional components and sheer timescale involved in sitting with a dying person. Doctors pop in and see bits of the process, and are divorced emotionally by their training and the need to fight off the inevitable, i.e. to *do* something, so that they cannot just *"be there for someone"*. That may change as a doctor actually experiences death (of a relative) in his or her own life. Remember all we can offer in most situations is our own humanity, and *never underestimate the value of this.*

Most of the comments in this chapter apply to death in later life or from chronic illness, rather than acute accidents or illnesses occurring in younger people, when every medical effort, however agonising to the patient, and it will be, should be attempted as a short-term measure.

Most people would like to die at home, in peace and surrounded or visited by friends and family, rather than hooked up to an obscene collection of tubes and drips in the regimented atmosphere of hospital. Dying at home takes practical organisational skills and at least one reliable relative or friend who will say "no" to calling 999/911 in any crisis, and requires the avoidance of hospitals and emergency services.

Planning death at home should probably start in ones 60s with consideration of the house, although the spiritual aspects of ones belief system about death should have been tackled earlier with books and suitable discussion. Since longevity (and illness) may run in families, looking at ones predecessors' ages at the time of death may give useful pointers. The house should contain at least one spare bedroom for use by a carer, later on, and should be sufficiently adaptable in case a downstairs bedroom and bathroom facility is needed. Falls are to be avoided at all costs. Broken bones mean hospital, incapacity and surrender of control to doctors.

If possible, one may employ someone younger as house-keeper or part time cook/shopper at an early stage, with a view to this person taking on a more personal role as needed later on. The alternative is to use nursing or carer agencies as required.

Make a will with advice from a solicitor, copies should be in an agreed place in the house, secure but easily unlocked when needed. One thing you can do to help your relatives avoid a great deal of grief and tears is to leave *written details of your own funeral service.* This includes whether burial or cremation, and where, and also the actual details of the service, choice of hymns, prayers, readings and music. (A local priest would help with this.) If an article has been written about your life then a copy of this would help the person writing the address (eulogy) who may not know details of your early life.

Most of the advice in this chapter comes from my own sad and fairly recent experience of the life and death (at 98, peacefully at home) of my Mother, which taught me far more about the process of dying than did my medical training. We were able to discuss her wishes many times.

The person concerned should be prepared for an "attack" of some sort, including illness and falls in public. If in pain, have someone search for medication (it does not matter what) in ones handbag (angina sprays are ideal), and then ask them to go and make tea. Don't let them near a telephone, people feel inadequate, and when they don't know what to do they dial 999, so keep them busy and take control if possible. (Say that it has all happened before.)

Some Advice for the Family at this Painful Time

Eventually the time will come when the person concerned wants to die, they should stay in bed (encourages pneumonia which used to be known as the old man's friend), stop eating and drink as little as possible, and

104

not take antibiotics. They should have told responsible relatives or friends of their wishes and have the carer, mentioned above, look after the details.

Friends and family can not sit with the dying all the time, many people die in the odd moment one slipped out for something. Do not feel guilty about this, some people may prefer to die alone, and may have chosen that moment. On a practical note, get a wireless baby alarm and leave the "baby" unit with the dying person, close enough so that you can hear their breathing via the receiving station unit downstairs, that way you can make meals etc. and would be aware if the breathing stops.

Organ Donation

These are my personal opinions, and I am "over 50" but you must make up your own mind for yourself. I would not be an organ donor (or recipient) for these reasons:

1   Death is a process, and we do not know if all the paraphernalia involved in life support machines and their eventual switching off, will interrupt this process, one would not wish to become an "arrested spirit" stuck here for eternity, haunting some benighted hospital corridor.

2   There is anecdotal evidence in the medical profession about what occurs when the apparently "brain dead" (tests done) donor's body is cut into in order to "harvest" (terrible euphemism) the organs. The donor's body must be kept oxygenated in order to maintain the organs to be "harvested" in good order, until the surgeons are ready with the recipient. Then the donor's body is cut into, without anaesthesia (he/ she is supposedly "brain dead") and the vital signs (pulse, blood pressure etc.) are visible to all in the theatre on monitor screens. At this point the blood pressure and pulse rate are seen to rise very considerably, and we must ask whether those diagnosed as "brain dead" *really do not feel pain?* We shall never know for sure.

Organ Donation Cards

At present the law says that those willing to donate may carry cards stating this. In view of the shortage of organs for donation (and demand will always exceed supply) there are suggested moves to take organs from anyone who has not specifically opted out. I personally carry a homemade wallet card stating that "for ethical reasons" I am not willing to be a donor.

I have great sympathy for those needing organ donation for life-threatening illnesses and the terrible dilemma of their families, especially where children are involved. However I do question the ethics of some of the more radical surgical procedures to which my profession is prepared to subject people, including in vitro fertilization and *selection* of embryos in order to use their cord blood cells or bone marrow to treat an older sick child.

As far as being a recipient goes, it is worth reading Paul Pearsalls fascinating book "The Heart's Code," which describes how people receiving heart transplants have had their tastes and outlook on life changed towards the personal tastes of their donor, *whom they did not know.* One little girl, who received the heart of another youngster who had been raped and murdered, started to suffer nightmares and flashbacks of the rape and murder. She required counselling to get over the "experience" but from her description, the police were able to catch the murderer. There are a number of other stories in this vein, and it gives one pause.

Afterword

Do not stand by my grave and weep,
I am not there I do not sleep.

I am the thousand winds that blow
I am the diamond glints on the snow.
I am the sunlight on ripened grain,
I am the gentle autumn rain.

When you waken in the morning's hush
I am the uplifting rush
Of quiet birds in circled flight.
I am the soft stars that shine at night.

Do not stand at my grave and cry,
I am not there I did not die.

by Unknown Author

Chapter 16

Electronic Medicine
The Pharmacy of the Future?

Having described some harmful effects of electricity in an earlier chapter, it is time to look at its healing and pain-relieving qualities. There are some electronic gadgets available through the internet at reasonable prices, which are effective and without side-effects. I will divide these into three groups, although there is an overlap as some machines do more than one thing. Most of the information in this chapter can be amplified by reference to the websites mentioned where there is much excellent original work. No scientific claims are made for these comments, but there are many anecdotal accounts of improvements of intractable illnesses, and no vast vested interests with major mercenary agendas. It is noteworthy that these machines are in such demand that they are often (temporarily) sold out.

Pain Relief

TENS Machines (Trans-cutaneous Nerve Stimulation)

There is a variety of these on the market – the best are small and portable. They consist of two or four electrodes placed on the skin near the painful area, and are connected by wires to a box supplying a suitable electric current through the electrodes. They certainly help.

Russian Skenar and Kosmed

These rather expensive machines are a result of the Russian space satellite programme in which scientists searched for an electronic pharmacy for the astronauts' illnesses as there were no facilities for drug use, and urine was being recycled. Some clever machinery was developed which had an element of bio-feedback, so that the machine could deliver the current and frequency required for the particular complaint. I am aware of problems in obtaining these machines and some of the instructions are so poorly translated that it is difficult to use them effectively. If the patent ever comes off so that this equipment becomes generally affordable and the above problems are solved, they may prove very useful. At present they are expensive to rent and not available for purchase.

Medicure

A magnetic device about the size of a pack of cards, this has three different frequencies for different purposes and is quite effective as a pain reliever, it also helps insomnia and several other complaints. It comes with an excellent Velcro bandage for attachment to the painful part. Reasonably priced.

Devices to Deal with Parasites and Infections

There is a school of thought in parts of the alternative medicine field, that much ill-health is caused by the presence of parasites including viruses, candida, yeasts, moulds and bacteria as well as flukes, worms and other unthinkables. It is suggested that we all carry about two and half pounds weight of parasites in our bodies … don't ask. Conventional medical tests for parasites are not very effective, stool specimens have to be very fresh and parasitology is not a popular branch of medicine, so it is possible that many of the tests that are carried out are falsely negative, and of course moulds, yeasts and viruses are not routinely tested for except in very limited bodily locations.

Further research on this subject should be pursued on the Internet through www.toolsforhealing.com who have an excellent description of the Beck Protocol and the work of Hulda Clark.

The Zapper has been updated and made easier to use, the Super Zapper Deluxe from www.toolsforhealing.com now comes with a selection of programme drivers which provide particular frequencies for treating different illnesses, and is very effective.

The Beck Protocol

This is a multi-pronged approach to the elimination of parasites, moulds yeasts and viruses using electrical devices for purifying the blood; ozonated water and colloidal silver which have antibacterial and antiviral properties.

The equipment includes the Silver Pulsar which is dual purpose and as well as making colloidal silver by electrolysis from distilled water, can be attached to ones wrist by two electrodes and the small current passed apparently acts as a blood purifier. The Magnetic Pulsar is a separate machine which is designed to kill parasites lurking in the lymphatic system, which would be missed by the blood purification process of the Silver Pulsar, it is an electromagnetic device which can be held over painful joints as it has pain relieving properties; or over lymph nodes.

The Beck Protocol also suggests the use of ozonated water to drink, (the extra oxygen atom has disinfecting properties). Incidentally ozone has had an unjustifiably bad press in connection with air pollution, although unencumbered with toxic gas emissions, it can be very beneficial as a sterilising agent. (See article on ozone on www.toolsforhealing.com, ozone has a long history of beneficial use in medicine. The website also sells an affordable water ozonator.)

Combined with these, one can use a Zapper, as designed by Hulda Clark, which also kills parasites electrically, but by a different mechanism. There are various designs of Zapper apart from the Super Zapper mentioned above, with different claims made for them. One of the easiest to use is the Terminator (www.elixa.com) in which the electrodes are attached to the machine, a very small box, which can be worn for long periods, unobtrusively under clothing. (Hint: stick the rough side of self-adhesive Velcro to the opposite side from the electrodes, and it will stay put.)

Brain Chemicals and Electronic Devices

There is a variety of devices designed to improve the way we feel by changing our brain chemicals or stimulating alpha waves (or both.) Here are two that I have used, a search of the internet reveals many more.

Brain Tuner

This is simple, portable and effective. It consists of a lightweight head set designed to go *behind* the ears, and make electrical contact with the skin, the headset is attached by wire to a small control box providing a choice of six different frequencies and modes of electrical stimulation, which can be comfortably felt over the skin behind the ears. It has automatic shut off after 20 minutes and should be used twice daily. (It is a development of the "black box" treatment for detoxifying drug addicts, pioneered by Meg Pattison in the early 1980s.) It probably works by stimulating brain chemicals (endorphins) which counter depression, and is not addictive. (Apparently over-use is counter-productive and will *reduce* the good effect, a case of "more *not* being better".) The machine can be used while doing household chores but not while driving a car. (www.toolsforhealing.com)

Proteus

This is a "light/sound" machine and works by a different process. It encourages brain wave frequency changes by entrainment to the light and sound frequencies chosen. There are several varieties of these machines and they all work on similar principles having a headset for the sound and a pair of specialised glasses which are equipped with light emitting diodes (little bulbs which light up and flash, usually red/green and are visible through the lids with the eyes shut). The headset and glasses are linked by wire to a small computer box which has various programmes and choices depending on whether stimulation, relaxation, learning or lucid dreams are the main requirement. There is considerable science behind this, more information can be found under "biofeedback" on the Internet (although most of the cheaper machines do not actually provide true biofeedback). By their nature, light/sound machines must be used sitting or lying down.

The Proteus machine (from www.elixa.com) is small and compact and can be used on long haul flights*. It has fifty pre-set programmes designed for different purposes and is reasonably simple to use, with options for choosing your own preferred frequency and light sequence, which it will memorise for future use. It also has possibilities for designing your own programmes, but this is only for those with an honours degree in computer engineering and a lot of time.

One must experience these machines first hand. They can produce indescribable bliss, and occasionally, out of body experiences. The only caveat is that those with forgotten, unresolved child abuse issues may start recalling things and require therapy. Both Proteus and Brain Tuner may increase dreaming.

---

* Since the heightened security fears following 9/11, it would be sensible to explain what the machine is to a cabin crew member. The flashing lights are visible to other people as reflections on the aircraft ceiling.

Seasonal Affective Disorder SAD

SAD is a depressive illness affecting some people who live in latitudes where there are short hours of daylight in the winter, and the sunlight is weak. It is seasonal and can be severe. The syndrome is related to lack of light reaching a part of the brain which regulates the production of melatonin, a sleep hormone. In these people, during the long winter months there is an overproduction of melatonin in the daytime with the resultant depression, carbohydrate craving and other symptoms. Some people have this problem so badly that, without treatment, it is incapacitating. Others and there are many, seem to get depressed and unhappy by mid-January in our latitude. They may also benefit from the treatment measures below.

Symptoms Include:
- Difficulty waking up in the morning
- Overeating carbohydrates and weight gain
- Depression, anxiety, energy loss and feeling of inability to cope
- Lowered resistance to infection.

Symptoms occur in winter and miraculously disappear around April.

Treatment

Lightboxes
SAD can be treated with full spectrum light boxes (from Healthy House among others). These provide bright light and this will stop the excess melatonin formation. Lightboxes are available in various brightnesses (measured in lux) and the brighter the light the more it costs and the less exposure time per day is needed. In general one needs to sit in front of the light daily for one to two hours, but can read, watch TV, computer etc. during this time.

The best time to use a lightbox is in the morning, and it should be avoided near bedtime as insomnia may result. Tinted or other glasses which change colour with light should not be worn as they negate the whole process. Changing the light bulbs in the house for full spectrum lights will not have the same effect as they are not bright enough.

Dawn Simulators
These are specialised alarm clocks which wake the sleeper by producing

an artificial dawn, the light bulb gradually illuminates from nothing to full daylight over 30 minutes at a preset time. (A buzzer can also be used for security, but most people disable it after a few days.) It is a way of waking gradually rather than being shattered by an alarm clock. The downside is that these clocks are relatively expensive but they double as a reading lamp, and will also do a dusk simulation which may help those with difficulty in going off to sleep (p129).

Chapter 17

European Food Supplements Directive

The European Parliament (for reasons given as safety and harmonisation) has decided to ban a large number of health foods, including minerals, vitamins, herbs and homeopathic preparations which can currently be purchased at heath food shops. Those vitamins and minerals allowed will be in a dosage too small to be of much use, and will be limited to a few choices (presumably chemically made by the big drug companies).

Many of the specialist health food companies have formulated products which are designed to be effectively absorbed (calcium, zinc) or not to cause diarrhoea (magnesium) for example; or to overcome other specific problems of which the non-specialist concerns have no experience. This law now applies in the EU, and may go through the British Parliament.

The history of this EU Law is obscure but used an (aptly named) piece of legislation called PARNUTS, involving cheap ingredients that may be added to food, to attempt to restore it to minimum nutritional value after the processors had removed all the original goodness in the processing (euphemistically called "adding value" but really meaning increasing the price.)

I have information that the real reason so many health foods, herbs and supplements are to be banned or only supplied in inadequately low dose, is related to behind the scenes lobbying by the big drug companies, who will be the beneficiaries if people are unable to obtain vitamins and minerals etc. in order to stay healthy, or to recover from environmental illnesses and problems related to nutritional deficiencies.

Modern agriculture has so degraded the land and our food that its mineral content is reduced, we should therefore be taking mineral supplements. If mineral intake is adequate, the body may cope with vitamin shortages, but without adequate minerals we get ill.

The reason given for this draconian measure is said to be "safety" and the idea is to ban any substance that has not been in use for 30 years or/ and undergone clinical trials to show its safety. Most of the products concerned are cheap and unpatented and would cost thousands of pounds each to test "double blind". There just isn't the money in it to justify the costs.

In general, I have come to the view that double blind clinical trials, funded by companies with an interest in the resulting expensive drug, are not to be relied upon, anyway. How can "he who pays the piper, not call the tune?" Very few people have died or been admitted to hospital from side effects of the products this directive seeks to ban, whereas the statistics for pharmaceuticals are horrific in this respect. (You are more likely to be struck by lightening than suffer ill health from taking food supplements.)

Cannabis (a herb) has just been decriminalised, tobacco (another herb) and alcohol (from the grape) all remain available for us to kill ourselves with; what possible benefit can this directive have other than to the vested interests concerned? It will criminalise people trying to stay healthy by natural means, who presumably will have to find a black market "pusher" from whom to buy their "substances". (Will "possession" be an offence? Presumably prescribing these items will?)

Where do herbal teabags stand (or soak) in all this? Homeopathic remedies will certainly be "off" and they are so dilute as not to have side-effects (let alone cause deaths). In fact, one of the gripes of the sceptics who debunk homeopathy is that the substances are so dilute that there is so little of the original ingredient in them that they can't possibly work. How then can they be "dangerous" other than to their competitors' share price?

The use of the spice Turmeric for the relief of arthritis pain is an interesting case in point. Currently it can be purchased from Lamberts in a concentrated tablet form, which is convenient to take and free of any side effects. If this is banned, we will still presumably be able to purchase Turmeric in powder form at the supermarket (weaker and much less convenient). Will there then be checks (by the "alternative substance police") to ensure that it is being used to make curry and not to treat arthritis? The Ministry of Stealth and Total Obscurity is fast becoming a reality.

This directive is being foisted on us at a time when the public is turning to alternative products because they are becoming increasingly dissatisfied with the drug-firm orientated "chemical solutions to human problems" approach to medicine, with all its expensive failings.

Enquiries reveal that this directive has already passed into EU Law, and that cannot be changed. We can still persuade our MPs not to pass this law in our Parliament by writing to them.

Enquiries also reveal that nobody knows exactly which products will be banned. I have a long list of those "ingredients" that will be proscribed, but

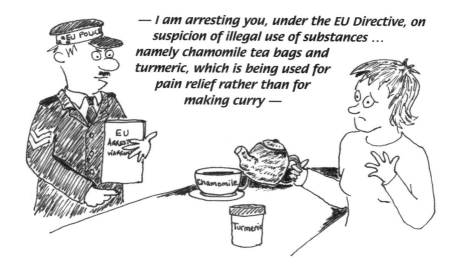

— I am arresting you, under the EU Directive, on suspicion of illegal use of substances ... namely chamomile tea bags and turmeric, which is being used for pain relief rather than for making curry —

a lot of decisions have not yet been made public, and as the time span is short, it seems amazing that we are not being told the truth, in advance.

More information can be obtained on this from Consumers for Health Choice (020 7222 4182.)

Postscript to this Chapter of Insanity:

In the USA during the late 1980s and early 90s, at least 80 people died and a further unknown number suffered a severe and disabling illness which became known as Eosinophilia-Myalgia Syndrome (EMS). This was eventually tracked down to a food supplement called L-tryptophan which had not previously caused problems. Medical detective work revealed that this illness occurred only in those who had taken a new variant of L-tryptophan made by Japanese drug company Showa Denko, which was produced using *genetically modified* ingredients.

All versions of L-tryptophan have been taken off the market.

It is becoming very clear that the genetic modifiers do not really know what they are doing, and can not replicate their products exactly, nor be sure of the contents of *each batch they make.*

Chapter 18

Alternative Pharmacy and Home First Aid Kit

*Items starred can be kept at home or taken on holiday as an "Alternative First Aid Kit".

Many of theses of commonly used alternative health products may become unavailable and/or illegal following introduction of the European Food Standards Directive, currently all can be bought in shops or by mail order.

Anti-Bacterial, Anti-Viral and Anti-Candida
- Colloidal Silver*
- Monolaurin*
- Oregano oil combinations
- Garlic Capsules
- Homeopathic Anas Barb 200*
  (Combinations of some of the above can reduce a cold from 5 weeks to five days and prevent a lot of infections)
- Olive leaf extract
- Citricidin and similar products
- Capricin and caprillic acid derivatives

Anti Parasitic
- Cloves
- Wormwood
- Black Walnut Hulls

Anti Allergy/Depression
- St John's Wort
- Boswelia herbal mixes

Immune System and General Boosters
- Evening Primrose Oil

- Cod liver oil
- Echinacea*
- Golden seal
- **Vitamins** in adequate dosage
- **Minerals** including Magnesium, Selenium and Zinc in an absorbable form

Gut Bacteria Improvers
- Acidophilus, lacto bacilli, variations on this. (Vital if taking antibiotics)
- Charcoal

Arthritis and Joint Pains (Anti-Inflammatory)
- Turmeric
- Boswellin
- White willow bark
- Chondroitin
- Glucosamine
- Homeopathic Rus. Tox, Ruta Grau, Arnica* and all homeopathic remedies.

Raised Blood Pressure
- Hawthorn

Stress and Anxiety
- Kava Kava (herb) this may be difficult to get and should be for short-term use.

Injury, Bruising and Surgery including Dentistry
- Homeopathic Arnica 30* which can be bought at larger chemists, is a miracle worker if used just before and immediately after surgery or dentistry, or as soon as possible after injury. No household should be without it.

Chapter 19

Practical Solutions to Common Problems

Unpleasant reactions to Vitamin and Herbal Products

Some people may find that certain vitamin or herbal preparations cause unwanted effects when swallowed (energy loss, cold shakes, depression etc.). Sometimes these problems can be prevented by taking the powder out of the capsule onto a spoon and carefully placing it *under* the tongue and allowing it to dissolve slowly. It is then absorbed directly into the system through the veins under the tongue and avoids the passage through the liver. I can not explain why this works but it usually does. If however this does not stop the ill-effects, I consider that the remedy is not suitable, and that the body is rejecting it for a reason.

Those who tend to react badly should start a new remedy when they can be at home for a few hours, and chose a time away from food (to avoid confusion with a food allergy reaction). The first (trial) dose should be a small amount (either one third of a pill, or a little powder taken out of the capsule) and swallowed with water and the time noted. If side effects have not occurred in about one hour they probably won't, and the item can be used normally.

If side effects do occur then a similar process can be tried using the trial dose placed under the tongue and not swallowed. If this trial is uneventful, then the item can be used in the dosage directed, provided it is dissolved under the tongue. This method requires organisation, as the dose may have to be divided, and must be taken away from meal times and conversation. If the substance still produces side effects, it should not be used.

Insomnia

Play a taped book or speech radio programme such as BBC Radio 4 or BBC World Service quietly, either through speakers, pillow-phone or floppy style headset. This works on the basis of "Mummy read me a story," with children, and is most effective if the material on the tape is familiar. Music does not work as well.

Health Pax from Elixa.com (phone 00 1505 293 4648, USA) is a small portable Cranial Electrical Stimulator consisting of electrodes which clip onto the earlobes, connected by leads to a control box which applies a suitable alternating current. This changes the brain wave frequency and encourages relaxation. Unofficial claims include improvement in anxiety, depression and insomnia after about three weeks regular use. It can be worn on aircraft for fearful fliers or round the house while doing other things. (But not while driving a car, operating machinery or trying to go to sleep.)

Recurrent Nightmares

These often follow trauma in childhood or more recent assault. They may be horrific and embarrassing in content. **Find a Dream Workshop** in another town, discuss the content of the nightmare(s), and if possible do a re-enactment of the dream with others from the group playing various parts as required. Try to build into the scenario a point at which you *become aware (in the dream) that you are dreaming*, this awareness enables you to take control of the dream action and/or wake up. Thank everyone involved in the workshop afterwards, but it is not necessary ever to meet them again. Somehow breaking the taboo and regaining the awareness, seems to reduce or eliminate the nightmares.

Drugs which cause nightmares in *some* people include Baclofen (a muscle relaxant), mefloquine (anti-malarial) and levo dopa derivatives sometimes used in Parkinsonism. Anyone suffering a sudden onset of nightmares after starting these or any other new medication, should ask their GP for an alternative.

Hauntings of People or Houses

Houses: The British Society of Dowsers (p128) keeps a list of members who specialise in dealing with this problem in a non-religious way. Most use plans or maps of the house and carry out absent healing, some come on site. One should send or offer a suitable "donation" as good dowsers often do not charge fees for ethical reasons.

People: Some dowsers also deal with hauntings that involve people, rather than houses, as do those involved with Personal Clearance (www.ericdowsett.com) who have a network of trained workers who do this work in different countries. An alternative is to approach the local church and ask for the Diocesan Exorcist, who should have experience of a religious approach.

Infections including Candida, Parasites and Chronic Ill Health

The terminator (Magnetic Zapper) from www.elixa.com is a neat modification Hulda Clarke's Zapper and uses copper electrodes placed directly onto the skin, and it can be worn under clothing as needed. Unofficial claims suggest that the current disrupts the cell walls of bacteria, yeasts, moulds and parasites which kills them. It can be combined with:

Colloidal Silver which is unofficially claimed to kill all the above infective organisms *without side effects* and can be used on a long-term basis. It works both internally and on the skin, on wounds etc. including a spray version for sinuses. I suspect it works better for some people than others and may not be a universal cure-all. It is expensive.

Natural Hormone Replacement Therapy (HRT)

Kinnard's Pharmacy, Sarasota, Florida, Tel: (USA) 001 942 366 0880 (www.kinnardspharmacy.com) supply natural HRT cream. They can arrange a saliva test to measure the levels of the various hormones and then make up the cream to suit the client's needs based on the test results.

Advantages: probably less damaging and more natural than other HRT in that the molecules used are closer to, or identical with, human hormones. Progesterone alone can be used, avoiding some of the problems of oestrogens, while still helping to preserve bone density.

Disadvantage: the saliva test is expensive, and the cream must be obtained by mail and paid for. You will need a doctor's assessment and prescription. I am prepared to do this, but it adds to the cost. Not available on the NHS.

If using this in our relatively cold climate, it is worth asking the pharmacy to make up the cream "double strength" and then use half the amount, otherwise one is left with acres of freezing exposed bare flesh while waiting for the cream to sink in.

Healing the Energetic Field (or Aura)

Gentle Wind Project, Kittery, Maine, Tel: (USA) 001 207 439 7639. www.gentlewind project.org

It is generally agreed that we are surrounded by an energy field, which may vary in size and integrity (some people see it as layers of fine mesh that may go into holes,) depending on our health and any past physical or emotional damage such as rape or other abuse. It probably gets damaged in the course of education and life in general. The Gentle Wind Project supplies healing instruments and runs seminars on this subject. Many dowsers also have healing approaches to the energetic field.

Minerals

It is true that, thanks to industrial farming, our food no longer contains the minerals that it should, and we would probably all benefit from effective mineral supplements, provided it is are in a *form that the body can absorb.* Some vitamin shortages can be withstood if we have adequate minerals, although it is a good idea to take a multivitamin too. Many minerals are supplied in pill form and travel unchanged through the intestine and straight down the loo. (Tablets should be chewed, and capsules opened or chewed in an effort to prevent this expensive waste.)

The mineral supplement which I recommend is a liquid called "Logic" from The Health Company Europe Ltd (www.thehealthcompany.tv). It tastes dreadful, and is improved minimally by mixing it with fruit juice or mineral water. Boots "Sprayvit" can be sprayed directly into the mouth for quick absorbtion.

Germanium Sesquioxide

This is a trace mineral which seems to have health benefits. It is not available in the UK but can be obtained from www.provitaminas.com in the USA. From personal experience it certainly helps with allergies, but so little research is available that I hesitate to recommend it. Germanium Sesquioxide was nearly banned in confusion with Germanium Oxide (a different product which has toxic effects on the kidneys) and the clinical trials appear to have been deliberately misleading, which made me wonder why anyone should bother to mislead us if Germanium Sesquioxide wasn't effective. A search of the internet reveals encouraging anecdotal information suggesting my observations may be right, and that it is a useful product.

Alternative Therapies for Arthritis and Joint Pain

Turmeric (a spice) and **Boswellin** (a herb from the tree that gives us the resin Frankincense) are helpful anti-inflammatories without serious side effects. **Chondroitin** is a powdered form of chicken cartilage and may help long-term. Gelatin can be used instead with the caveat that it is theoretically possible for it to transmit BSE. Either should be from an organic source.

Glucosamine (often combined with chondroitin) is very helpful for some people. I would add the proviso that I tried it and it made me feel very angry (for no reason) the next day, and this was so unpleasant that I avoid it scrupulously.

Therapeutic Use of Magnetism

There is a number of magnetic products on the market, from straps to waistcoats and wraps. It is now well accepted that magnets can be used to treat various conditions successfully, including musculo-skeletal disorders, such as backache, arthritis, acute and chronic injuries, cramp, some skin disorders. There is evidence from Russia that magneto-therapy may strengthen the immune system. It can also help with energy loss.

Adrenaline Sports (Appendix 2) make a magnetic waistcoat and various sized wraps for injured limbs, the wraps have one pocket for the magnet and another for a hot/cold pack; the combination works better than either alone.

The mechanism of magneto-therapy is unclear, but it undoubtedly reduces pain. There is a beneficial effect on potassium ions in the cells that have been damaged by injury or illness.

Alternative Pathology Laboratory

Biolab (0207 636 5959) in London carry out tests for mineral and vitamin deficiencies and overloads, using blood urine and sweat tests, they also have a range of other tests which are useful for those interested in avoiding the "pill fairy." They do require a doctor's request for these tests and the doctor should be able to interpret the results and advise the patient on subsequent action.

Postscript

Why I have Written this Book

Most authors have a hidden agenda. I do not, any more, want worldly "fame" (which is notoriety, and involves loss of privacy), nor did I write it primarily for money. I have no products to sell. I feel that through my life and particularly through the difficulties I have encountered on the journey, I have found some useful solutions that are worth passing on. My medical training has been helpful in this but only when combined with my experience as a human being on the journey of life. I have learned a great deal by listening to people and patients. So here are a few trite but useful sayings for you to take on your journey.

For doctors and health care workers:
* Don't listen to the doctor, listen to the patient.

For the rest of us:
* There are no solutions, all solutions create other problems. All important decisions must be made on inadequate information.

* The only thing we have to offer is our own humanity but never underestimate the value of this.

* Consider the lilies of the field, for they vacuum not, neither do they scrub (more often than absolutely necessary).

* Life is a bit like a toilet roll, the closer you get to the end, the faster it goes.

* Life is not "fair".

* The rain it raineth on the just and unjust fella
  But mainly on the just,
  For the unjust has pinched the just's umbrella.

Enjoy the journey …!

Appendix 1

Further Reading

Food

Seeds of Deception. Jeffrey M Smith. (Yes! Books ISBN 0-9729665-8-7.)

Genetically Engineered Food. Cummins and Littiston 2000. (Marlow & Co.)

Toxic Sludge is Good for You. Stauber & Rampton 1995 (Community Courage Press. Maine.)

Fast Food Nation. Eric Schlosser (Penguin.)

The Hay Diet:
Food Combining for Health. Grant & Joice. Thorsons.

Food Additives, a Shoppers Guide to What's Safe and What's Not. Christine Hoza Farlow. (Kiss for Health Publishing (USA) Tel: 001-760-7358101.)

Dinner at the New Gene Café. Bill Lambrecht. (ISBN 0-312-30263-0.)

A New Shoppers Guide to Organic Food. Lynda Brown. (Fourth Estate.)

The Cholesterol Myths. Uffe Ravnskov, MD, PhD. (New Trends Publishing Inc.)

The End of the Line. How Overfishing is Changing the World. Charles Clover 2004. Ebury Press.

The Journey of Life

Further Along the Road Less Travelled. M Scott Peck. (Simon and Schuster.)

People of the Lie. M Scott Peck. (Simon and Schuster.)

Rescuing Your Spirit. John Freil, PhD. (Health Communications Inc.)

Banished Knowledge. Alice Miller. (Anchor Books.)

Learning to Love Yourself. Sharon Wegscheider-Cruse. (Health Communications Inc.)

Healing Words. Larry Dossey MD. (Harper Paperbacks.)

Shadow World. Brad Steiger. (Penguin Putnam Inc.)

Adult Children. The Secrets of Dysfunctional Families. John Freil and Linda Freil. (Health Communications Inc.)

Sick Houses

Safe as Houses? David Cowan and Rodney Girdlestone. (Gateway Books.)

Healing Sick Houses. Roy and Ann Procter. (Gateway.)

Geopathic Stress. How Earth Energies affect our Lives. Jane Thurnell-Reid. (Element.)

Candida, Yeast infections

The Yeast Connection. William G Crook MD. (Thorsons)

Miscellaneous

Plague, Pestilence and the Pursuit of Power. Steven Ransom. (Credence Publications)

Dirty Medicine (out of print) Martin J Walker 1994. (Slingshott ISBN 0-9519646-0-7)

Dogs that Know when their Owners are Coming Home. Rupert Sheldrake, (ISBN 0-09-925587-1)

Appendix 2

Useful Information

Dr Diana Samways

01428 654850 (rapid message handling service.)

12 Step Self-help Groups

Alcoholics Anonymous 0845 769 7555.

Al-Anon and Ala-teen 0845 769 7555.

Cocaine Anonymous 020 7284 1123.

Co-dependents Anonymous 020 7376 8191. (Adult Children of Alcoholics and other family issues.)

Families Anonymous 020 7398 4680. (Relatives and friends of those with a drug problem.)

Gamblers Anonymous 020 7384 3040. (Compulsive gamblers, line shared with GamAnon, for their families or friends.)

Narcotics Anonymous 020 7730 0009. (Helpline 10am-10pm weekdays.)

Overeaters Anonymous 07000 784985. (Eating disorders including overeating, anorexia and bulimia)

Treatment Centre

Rehabilitaion for alcohol and drug problems, also eating disorders: Promis (Kent) 01304 841700 (Rehabilitation to abstinence, fee paying.)

Workshops for Adults suffering from the effects of Child Abuse

Don Lavender 01363 83937 (England.)

Sierra Tucson (Arizona) www.sierratucson.com

Caron Foundation (Pennsylvania) www.caron.org

(All fee paying but brief, weekend or a week.)

Charity running helpline and information for children of alcoholics and adults:

National Association for Children of Alcoholics (Bristol) 0117 924 8005

Alternative Blood and other Tests

Biolab Medical Unit. (Blood tests for vitamin deficiencies, toxic overloads and other problems.)
020 7636 5959/5905.

Immunotherapy (for food and inhalant allergies.)

McEwen Laboratories (E.P.D). Tel: 01491 576314. Dr L McEwen

Bughwood Clinic (Neutralisation Therapy) Tel: 01737 361177.

Other Support Groups:

Campaign for Freedom from Piped Music (in public places.) Pipedown 01980 623945.

The National Candida Society. www.candida-society.org.uk (01689-813039.)

Prozac Support Group and Psychiatric Reactions to Drugs: www.April.org.uk

Geopathic Stress and other Adverse House Energies:

British Society of Dowsers 01684 576969.

Elizabeth Brown 07974 918927.

House Energy Clearance www.ericdowsett.com

Electrical Phenomena: Power Watch www.powerwatch.org.uk

Location of Mobile Phone masts, by area: Sitefinder, www.sitefinder.radio.gov.uk

Useful Websites and Product Information

Journals and Publications

Greenhealthwatch 01309 611231.

The Food Commission (020 7837 2250) is an independently funded body that sells two excellent posters giving detailed information on food additives and decoding food labels and publishes The Food Magazine.

Weston A Price Foundation publish an excellent magazine called Wise Traditions (funded by subscription, not by the food industry.) www.westonaprice.org

Wessex Cancer Help Centre. 01243 778516. A Charity, publishes good information on alternative products in its newsletter.

Supplements:

Alternative Pharmacy
Nutri Centre 020 7637 8436 all supplements, herbs etc. including Monolaurin, Candigest.

Vitamin B spray for those allergic to other Vitamin B preparations: Sprayvit multivitamin from Boots.

Liquid Mineral Product: Logic 0870 2405501.

New alternative anti-fungal: Candigest and Candigest Plus. (Nutri Centre.)

Germanium Capsules: www.Provitaminas.com (USA.)

Natural Hormone Replacement Therapy
Kinnards Pharmacy, Sarasota, Florida. 001 941 366 0880. Oestrogen and progesterone creams, saliva tests.

Colloidal Silver
Julian Bing 01494-489014.

Homeopathic Pharmacy
Ainsworths 020 7935 5330.
Nelsons 020 7629 3113.

Suppliers of Equipment

Healthy House (Lightboxes, dawn simulators, Airfree and Nasalairguard) 01453 752216.

Natural Collection. (Airfree, Lightboxes, other equipment and environmentally friendly products.) 01225 404020.

Other Products and Websites

Air Purifiers, Light /Sound (Brainwave) Machines and other gadgets: www.elixa.com

Parasites, Beck Protocol and good Information, Zappers: www.toolsforhealing.com

Juicer: L'Equip Mini Pulp Ejector Juicer: www.lequip.com

Magnetic Wraps and Waistcoats: Adrenaline Sports Ltd. 0870 7706910.

Protection against Electrical and other Undesirable Frequencies: Neutralec Neutralisers and Personal Protection Discs. 01562 823824.

Steam Inhaler for Colds: Vicks (Kaz) 0117 930 0818.

Appendix 3

Translating Food Package Labelling

I can only offer brief hints. "Food Additives A Shopper's Guide to What's Safe & What's Not" is an excellent pocket guide for those in the USA. The situation in Europe is different and the Food Commission (0207 837 2250) an independently funded body has two excellent posters giving detailed information. A trawl through the internet on this subject is surprisingly unhelpful as many of the websites are sponsored by major players in the food industry, which may not be immediately obvious.

Basically it is a good idea to avoid foods which look like a chemist's paradise and have a long list of additives and chemicals. However this is not always possible so:

- Be aware that any beverage marked with a fruit (say orange) followed by the word *"drink"* contains very little of the fruit mentioned, instead it contains sugar, colouring, water and flavouring. Fruit *juice*, should contain fruit (plus preservatives, and any pesticides and moulds that came with the fruit). Caveat; manufacturers do not usually make fruit juice (or baby food) with best quality fruit, so either may have a mould count of its own.

- **Sugars**
  Anything ending in –ose or –ase is a sugar. The list includes sucrose, fructose, glucose, dextrose and high fructose corn syrup. Often sugars are broken down so they appear more than once on the list. In theory the most abundant chemical in the food appears first, and the rest in diminishing order by weight. By splitting the sugars, this can be obfuscated.

- **Salt**
  Usually appears with sugar. Both are cheap, and used together they are said to improve "mouth feel" (consistency). Some foods seem to consist almost entirely of these two ingredients (including supermarket prawn cocktail and some Chinese and Indian Dishes).

One can always tell, afterwards, as one will be incredibly thirsty a few hours later. I will *never* buy that product (or eat at that restaurant) *again*, so; food manufacturers, this is shortsighted and bad for profits. I call this the "salt and sugar game". It has nothing to do with nutrition and everything to do with profit.

- **Preservatives**
  Include ascorbic acid (which is vitamin C). Citric acid is synthetic lemon juice. Acetic Acid is synthetic vinegar. Many other products are used.

- **Added Synthetic Vitamins**
  In the USA synthetic B vitamins are added to most bread, rice and much else. They can cause allergic or other food reactions, and are marked on the packaging as Niacin, Thiamine, Biotin, etc. Their inclusion tells me that the product is heavily processed and to be avoided if possible. The manufacturers boost sales by advertising the "added vitamins" without mentioning that they were first processed out. Breakfast cereals in the UK are now being fortified in this way, presumably as a hook to suggest to parents that they are "healthy." Cereal packets are well worth a read, sugar in various forms ranks highly among ingredients listed as do chocolate and fats, in some cases.

- **Aspartame**
  Is an artificial sweetener to be avoided. It has not been adequately tested, and there is some evidence that it may cause nerve damage. Good quality honey, used in moderation is a much sounder approach to sugar restriction. "Sweet tooth" tends to diminish once one stops sweetening things with sugar.

This is a short list of the basic additives. It is a highly complex subject which should be further researched through books written by experts and *unbiased* websites. Many people are allergic to, or hyped up by, the artificial colouring and flavouring agents added to food and soft drinks.

Appendix 4

Entrainment of Brain Waves by Pulsed Signals

Dr Diana Samways MBBS

The TETRA system may have electrical effects that disrupt body functioning. This system is untried as a communications medium, but a similar inaudible pulsed signal of 11 – 25 cycles per second was used during the cold war to cause adverse behavioural changes in people, and it may also have caused some cases of leukaemia, long term.

As a doctor specialising in Allergy and Environmental Medicine, my concern is with the probable effects on brain function with respect to our brain waves, the small electrical signals our brain uses to control all our vital body functions, mood and our normal communications with each other. These small electrical "waves" can be seen and measured using head electrodes and an Electro-Encephalogram (EEG) machine. Normally our brainwaves "pulse" at frequencies between 1 and 40 cycles per second (cps) *depending on what we are doing*. TETRA "pulses" at 17.5 cps which is well in our Beta wave range (see diagram).

Certain frequencies of brainwaves occur in different states of consciousness. While we are awake and active Beta waves (14 - 20 cycles per sec.) predominate, but this is not peaceful, and has an element of chronic hurry about it. (Watch the crowd at any airport.)

Alpha waves (8 -13 cps) are associated with relaxation and meditation, and Theta waves (4 -7 cps) with deep meditation also creativity and inspiration and pre-sleep states, Delta waves (1 –4 cps) with deep sleep needed for restoration, healing and well being. In the scale of man made airwaves, our brainwaves are of small amplitude, i.e. relatively weak, which makes us vulnerable.

EEG Pattern	Name	Frequency	Psychological state
~~	Beta	14 - 40	Alert
ᴧᴧᴧᴧᴧᴧᴧᴧᴧᴧ	Alpha	8 - 13	Usually eyes closed, relaxed wakefulness
ᴧᴧᴧᴧᴧᴧᴧ	Theta	4 - 8	Hypnogogic state, early stages of sleep
ᴧᴧᴧᴧᴧ 50μV 1 sec	Delta	1 - 4	Deep sleep

The Relationship between Brainwave Frequency (in cycles per second), Electro-Encephalograph Tracing and State of Mind.

Diagram reprinted by permission of Dave Siever, C.E.T.,
from "Audio-Visual Entrainment Technology".

Entrainment of Brainwaves using Pulsed Signals (Flashing Lights, Music or other Signals)

We all know that combinations of flashing lights, and some music can be "mood altering" (the Mozart Effect, night clubs, pop bands etc.). This works by using the mechanism of Brain Wave Entrainment.

Entrainment is a phenomenon in which powerful rhythmic vibrations of one object will cause the less powerful vibrations of another object to lock in step and oscillate (pulse) at the first object's rate (frequency). It occurs throughout nature. For example if you have several similar pendulum clocks on a wall and start them in motion at different times, they will all swing differently. If you go away and come back next day, they will all be swinging together in phase. (Discovered by Dutch scientist Christian Huygens in 1665.)

Unlike resonance which is passive, entrainment seems to be active, and involves changing the natural oscillatory pattern of one object and replacing it with the different oscillatory pattern of another. People having an intimate conversation entrain their brain waves so that they are "in phase". Skilled public speakers entrain with their audience. Other examples include fireflies flashing in phase, the synchronisation of breathing in a group setting, and of menstrual cycles in enclosed orders after a period of time, so the nuns menstruate simultaneously.

This phenomenon can be applied clinically in the field of bio- and neuro-feedback training, which aims to alter the person's brainwave pattern so that they feel better and symptoms and behaviour improve. (Alpha frequencies are usually encouraged in neuro-feedback techniques.) Clearly the opposite would occur using the wrong frequencies.

It is likely that the brain will lock onto the signals from TETRA equipment (Beta at 17.5 cps, brain in work and hurry mode) and stay there, so that our normal functions of relaxation, creativity and sleep will be impaired or disrupted, leading to stress, mood swings, insomnia etc. and poor immune system function. (Reports of this are already being heard.)

In this respect the TETRA system differs from the existing mobile phone system, and it was this mechanism (using frequencies in the 11-25cps range) that was successfully used in the cold war to disrupt health and behaviour.

Copyright © Dr Diana Samways MBBS